Chapter 1

The Genesis

*"Where there's no struggle,
there's no strength."*
— Oprah Winfrey

1

Cancer is a sickness that has affected maximum humans's lives in a single manner or any other. If you haven't heard of a person being identified with most cancers, whether or not they're near you or now no longer, you've got got truly been residing beneathneath a rock! I jest, however it's far a reality of cutting-edge existence. Not simplest has my own circle of relatives been deeply impacted with the aid of using this sickness, I myself have as well. Unfortunately, I even have misplaced 5 own circle of relatives participants (nuclear and extended) to this sickness, and I myself acquired my personal most cancers prognosis. This sickness has continually been a part of my existence in a single manner or any other.

After my recuperation adventure from most cancers, I felt known as to percentage that adventure with you. I no longer simplest believe, however I understand for a reality, that this sickness does now no longer should be a loss of life sentence. I need to make certain that now no longer simplest my pals and own circle of relatives understand this however which you understand this as well. I need you now no longer to sense terrified of this killer lurking withinside the shadows. Instead, I need you to understand which you have many alternatives to be had to you so that you can start combating any opportunity of this sickness TODAY.

I need to percentage with you now no longer simplest my revel in in confronting most cancers head on, however what I discovered alongside the manner. Most humans sense that this sickness is some thing this is out in their control. But I am right here to inform you, it's far NOT. Cancer isn't always simplest conquerable, however it's far preventable in a myriad of ways. Throughout this ee-e book I will percentage the whole lot I discovered by myself adventure to curing my most cancers with out using conventional capsules or the standard western remedy direction of action. As you read, please bear in mind that I am now no longer a medical doctor or healer. I became in search of solutions and had a perception that there ought to be any other manner to manipulate this sickness that has ravaged many lives. I am right here to show that there's any other manner to be most cancers-unfastened and complete of vitality. I am satisfied you're right here, and wish my tale serves you and those you love.

The Start of My Journey

One of my mentors continually careworn to me: "If you preserve doing what you've got got continually done, you'll preserve ge&ng what you've got got continually got." So, whilst it got here to my most cancers prognosis, I explored the opportunity of doing some thing different. As I cited earlier than, this sickness had already determined its manner into my existence with the aid of using taking the lives of these I loved. So, all I noticed became a opportunity of taking any other avenue to coping with this sickness, as I became decided that it'd now no longer be the stop of existence. Furthermore, I desired to position an stop to the generational curse of dropping own circle of relatives participants from this deadly sickness.

Back in October 2014, one week earlier than visiting to Asia, I became running with a homeopathic medical doctor who ended up diagnosing my proper breast as "now no longer functioning well." Because I became withinside the procedure of visiting, I simply disregarded the notion, because it became now no longer a pinnacle precedence at that time. I do my breast self-examinations religiously and urge every body to do them! If you're of childbearing age, each girls AND guys must be doing those critical month-to-month self-assessments as mammograms aren't 100% accurate. Mammograms do now no longer hit upon all kinds of most cancers withinside the breast.

While I became residing withinside the USA, sooner or later I did sense a lump in my proper breast. I right away sought an opinion from my medical doctor who honestly stated that I had "dense breasts" and there has been not anything to fear approximately. I depended on the opinion of a clinical expert However of direction endured the exercise of doing self-examinations. After numerous years, having moved to Canada, I did once more sense a brand new form of lump in my breast. However, this time it felt different. I went returned to my medical doctor's opinion and honestly chalked it as much as the reality that I had "dense breasts" and did now no longer react to it right away. But after numerous months, I ought to sense that this lump grew in size, and this is whilst alarm bells went off in my mind. I knew in my intestine that this became greater than only a prognosis of "dense breast" tissue.

I right away booked an appointment with my own circle of relatives medical doctor. I shared what I had observed and, yes, they showed that I had a lump in my proper breast. I right away went in for a mammogram and ultrasound to get a
right prognosis of what became occurring in my body. The medical doctor's assistant known as me the subsequent morning and advised me the medical doctor desired to look me proper away. From the tone of her voice, I ought to inform that the information I became approximately to get hold of became now no longer going to be positive.

Diagnosis

I will in no way neglect about August 1, 2019. This is the day I turned into identified with breast most cancers. When the medical doctor instructed me the information, you can pay attention a pin drop. We had been each actually upset. They recorded an in depth account of my family's records with most cancers to benefit a higher expertise of what we had been up in opposition to. I turned into mentioned a pinnacle oncologist at one of the fine most cancers hospitals in Canada. We did all important exams aND once more I turned into given a nice breast most cancers prognosis. More in particular a Stage 2 prognosis, which shows that the sickness turned into detected in its early stages. Immediately my mind went to Dr. Debra Williams, ND. Dr Williams is a naturopathic medical doctor, and scientific missionary in Jamaica who additionally had Stage 2 breast most cancers and cured it with out chemotherapy. She have become my inspiration! I knew there has been mild on the give up of the tunnel.

I opted now no longer to have a mastectomy (a surgical treatment to take away a breast) and selected the second one alternative of getting the lump eliminated and a sentinel node biopsy, so that it will decide if the most cancers had unfold to some other components of my frame. I turned into elated to research that it had now no longer! The subsequent step turned into to start rounds of chemotherapy, accompanied through radiation treatments. However, after gaining knowledge of the information that the lump had now no longer unfold, I boldly exercised my patient's invoice of rights and opted NOT to have chemotherapy. Of course, that is an uncommon pass that turned into now no longer taken gently through my oncologist. "I were an oncologist for twenty-5 years and none of my sufferers have ever refused chemotherapy treatment," he instructed me, perhaps withinside the wish that I could alternate my mind, or to make sure that I knew I turned into virtually going in opposition to the grain.

I did now no longer take this desire gently. But I turned into very sure. I remembered the words, "If you hold doing what you've got got continually done, you'll hold getting
what you've got got continually got" on this situation. I felt deep down that if I accompanied the traditional course it'd cause the equal destiny of my relatives: now no longer surviving this sickness.

I enlisted a holistic medical doctor to assist me with this new leg of my adventure, and stale we went. Fast ahead a 12 months later to August 2020, after I had a follow-up breast ultrasound and mammogram with my oncologist. He tested my proper breast and exclaimed, "Whatever that medical doctor did to you, she or he did an excellent job!" I couldn't assist however smile like a Cheshire cat! It has now been over 2 years for the reason that my most cancers prognosis and I am glad to document that my breast most cancers stays in remission.

Now which you have a picture of my complete most cancers story, I am searching ahead to diving into a few paintings with you. I need to proportion with you the entirety I discovered in this adventure that took me from the opportunity of living (or dying) with a sickness to being most cancers-free. Today I sense I am withinside the fine fitness I actually have ever been, and I want that for you and your family as well. Whether you're preventing the sickness now or simply need to have in mind and stay in a extra preventable way, I need to reveal you that super fitness is offered irrespective of from in which you're beginning. Let us dive in!

Setting Yourself Up and Starting From Where You Are

If you're ever to stand adversity, be it a warfare with most cancers or some thing else, you need to set your self up proper to virtually have the energy to fight. Of course, there's a bodily energy component. However, maximum of what you want to harness is the intellectual energy to face up to this warfare. It may be an extended and hard adventure to regain your complete fitness. At the give up of the day, it comes right all the way down to having the right attitude.

I need to proportion with you a few beginning factors to benefit angle on what I evolved after which took with me at some stage in my adventure. The maximum essential component on this second is to keep in mind to begin from in which you're. Start precisely from anything attitude and intellectual mindset you've got got and emerge as dedicated to increasing that to be the fine you may be.

Positive Mental Attitude

"Two guys seemed out from jail bars; one noticed mud, the alternative noticed stars."

- Dale Carnegie

I sense this quote flawlessly depicts how I turned into feeling at some stage in my most cancers adventure, specially after I turned into first identified. Having most cancers made me sense like I turned into a prisoner. A prisoner to my frame and this prognosis. Suddenly my existence turned into diagnosed in a exclusive mild. However, simply because the prisoner who seemed out of the jail mobileular and noticed stars, I turned into hopeful.

Someone near me turned into additionally going via his very own most cancers struggle on the time. He gave me the pleasant recommendation while he cautioned me to live hopeful, irrespective of what, as it'd assist with my restoration procedure. That first piece of recommendation turned into invaluable, specifically understanding what I recognise now. A restoration procedure rooted in desire is critical while going through this ailment. Hope is one thing of getting a fantastic intellectual mindset.

Positive intellectual mindset (PMA) is a idea first delivered via way of means of Napoleon Hill in 1937 withinside the famous book, Think and Grow Rich. This idea has seeing that been followed via way of means of many that need to create alternate of their lifestyles. When you've got got the proper intellectual mindset in any situation, it draws fantastic alternate and outcomes on your lifestyles. Having a evolved and sturdy PMA is critical while coping with most cancers.

Studies had been performed which genuinely display a correlation to sufferers having a sturdy fantastic intellectual mindset and getting better from infection faster, instead of sufferers who view lifestyles with a greater poor gaze. I can in reality attest to this personally. Not simplest did I actually have my very own evolved feel of positivity, I turned into additionally surrounded via way of means of fantastic support. I actually have heat recollections of my siblings sending me vegetation and playing cards to reveal their support. I favored those type gestures greater than they may imagine. When I noticed their gifts, I turned into usually reminded to return back again to a fantastic area in my thoughts.

Starting from in which you're, do you sense which you bring a fantastic mind-set or do you generally tend to stay in a greater poor kingdom? Wherever you're at, even in case you sense you're commonly a fantastic person, it's far usually a terrific concept to preserve to domesticate a fantastic intellectual mindset within. This will allow you to preserve for your journey, whether or not it's far combating ailment or some thing else lifestyles throws at you, with top notch desire.

Visualizations

Visualizations are a totally effective device that you could use for many stuff on your lifestyles.

You can also additionally have already heard approximately the usage of visualizations on your lifestyles. During the adventure of restoration my most cancers, I might harness the electricity of visualization and spot myself being healed and most cancers-unfastened in my thoughts's eye a couple of instances a day. This saved me stimulated and driven, and additionally acted as a guiding put up for my frame. Through visualizing that I turned into healthy, I gave unconscious thoughts and steering to my frame. I turned into directing it to the kingdom I desired it to be in: most cancers-unfastened!

Beyond visualizing together along with your thoughts, there are different techniques, including growing a imaginative and prescient or dream board. A imaginative and prescient board is a group of pix, words, terms and colors, both assembled altogether onto one board or genuinely pinned for my part onto a board. The pix constitute what you need to BE, DO and HAVE. You create a photo of your future. It is a laugh to have pix pinned one at a time on a board so you can switch them to a "completion" board if you have performed them. Another top notch visualization device is to have your desires written on man or woman playing cards that you could study all through the day. These playing cards are without difficulty portable and may assist hold your thoughts centered on aligning together along with your desires.

As you could see, that is a effective all-spherical device to apply to your lifestyles. When you're the usage of visualization to enhance your fitness or rid your self of a ailment as I turned into the usage of it, it turns into any other vital piece of a bigger puzzle with the intention to assist lead you to heal your frame and create higher fitness.

Affirmations

In addition to visualizations, many a hit humans additionally use affirmations as a part of their day by day practices that hold them in a fantastic mind-set and set themselves up for greatness. Before my most cancers diagnosis, I already had a day by day exercise of each visualizations and affirmations, so I felt a chunk greater organized once I had to pivot the center reason.

Affirmations are sayings or fees which you recite to your self each day so that it will increase your fantastic energy. They create an possibility with the intention to connect with mind and emotions that make you sense good, or feeling higher than you presently do.

I need to proportion with you a number of my favourite affirmations which have truly helped me. They hold me feeling fantastic and grounded. During my struggle with most cancers, I welcomed them into my lifestyles wholeheartedly:

- I praise you because I am fearfully and wonderfully made. (Psalm 13 NIV
- I trust you wholeheartedly and surrender my life to your guidance.
- God grant me the strength to change what I can, the courage to accept I can't, and wisdom to know the difference. (Serenity Prayer)
- I am open to receiving. I remain patient, positive, loving and faithful.

Do you've got got any affirmations that encourage you? You might also additionally have one or several. They might also additionally come from exclusive reassets or humans. The maximum critical issue is that whilst you recite them, they make you experience alive, hopeful and geared up to conquer any adversity you will be facing. Or they could surely act as a lift in your strength each day. If you presently do now no longer have any affirmations which you practice, I inspire you to discover at the least one that could serve you transferring forward!

Possible Causes of Cancer

The verbal exchange round what reasons most cancers is extensive. As I noted on this ee-e book, I may be discussing life-style picks that I located contributed at once to me taking my fitness again from this terrible disease. It is quite eye-establishing at how empowered we're whilst bringing ourselves to a high, superb nation of fitness. Beyond what I will talk approximately are some matters really well worth bringing up that I need to attract interest to. You can then pick to start your very own studies on those particular elements in case you wish.

Starting with analyzing your food plan is essential, and one of the first actual matters that you could do immediately. Do you consume plenty of processed meals or clean entire meals? I will move into element approximately ingredients I were consuming to live wholesome in addition to speak trendy amount and frequency of consuming in some other chapter. But permit me first plant a seed for your thoughts with the query I asked.

A few larger, extra vast subjects I will now no longer be overlaying extensive on this ee-e book as you could actually write complete books on positive most cancers-inflicting factors alone. I need to in short point out them, though, so you can in addition look at for your self.

The surroundings you stay in can at once have an effect on your fitness. You might not be aware about what number of pollution are genuinely surrounding you at any given moment. From transportation to agriculture to normal family activities, you're continuously uncovered to chemical compounds that have an effect on your fitness. You will by no means be capable of keep away from all of them together. However, whilst you start to recognize how massive of a scale that is, you could then deal with the matters that you could genuinely be capable of control (plenty of this is included on this ee-e book.) When it comes right all the way down to it, pollution aren't evidently taking place elements of your surroundings, so that they may be unfavourable in your fitness.

Genetics can play a element withinside the opportunity of having most cancers in some unspecified time in the future for your existence. Take myself for example. I trust that is how I ended up with breast most cancers. As I noted in my dedication, I even have had 5 humans in my own circle of relatives die due to the disease. So in hindsight it does now no longer wonder me that I ended up with a most cancers diagnosis.

In our current international there's one issue this is very hard to break out: pressure! Stress can are available in many paperwork from minor to major, and may be visible as a completely massive a part of the various approaches your fitness can malfunction. It is multifaceted and may at instances be complicated. While you may maximum in all likelihood by no means be capable of genuinely break out pressure altogether, the important thing may be to manipulate it properly. Based on research that I study approximately thru City of Hope (www.cityofhope.org), continual pressure can initiate most cancers to unfold quicker (mainly in breast, colorectal and ovarian most cancers). Science says that once our our bodies grow to be worn-out and harassed out, neurotransmitters inclusive of norepinephrine (additionally a pressure hormone) are launched into the body, which stimulates most cancers cells. So believe in case you are continuously beneathneath a constant hum of pressure. Chronic pressure isn't anyt any joke, and it's far as much as you to recognize your pressure and discover ways to manipulate as quickly as possible. Your existence might also additionally depend upon it!

I am so thankful you're right here and looking to examine extra approximately my adventure. It manner you care approximately your self and your cherished ones, and trust withinside the opportunity of now no longer most effective being most cancers-free, however additionally trust in residing a wholesome and energized existence in trendy. The first a part of my recovery adventure become to extrade a few easy life-style picks that won't appear like a lot, however on the quit of the day absolutely are sport changers.

Chapter 2

Necessary Lifestyle Changes

"Change will now no longer come if we look forward to a few different character or a few different time. We are those we were ready for. We are the extrade that we seek."

— Barack Obama

2

I become off on my adventure to heal my frame and rid myself of breast most cancers. I determined to paintings carefully with a holistic physician who desired to create a focal point on converting components of my lifestyle that would be negatively contriButing to my health. We recognized the factors of my existence that wanted fundamental overhaul and a few that simply absolutely required a chunk of tweaking. Our aim become to alternate habits, enhance my health, after which permit myself to combat the most cancers in my frame. I will define a number of the primary adjustments I without difficulty carried out proper away. When I first carried out them, I of direction become doing it due to my diagnosis. But, pricey reader, you do now no longer ought to wait till you're unwell to tackle whatever I talk on this bankruptcy or past. I genuinely urge you to take the whole lot on this ee-e book to coronary heart and start to apprehend that there's some thing to be stated for preventative measures.

Personal Care Products

The first matters I need to study are the severa normal non-public care merchaNDise which are part of your grooming and hygiene routines. I guess that lots of you analyzing this may relate to the reality that you will be the use of extra traditional gadgets with out even a notion as to what's genuinely in those merchandise, not to mention how they're affecting your frame. My holistic physician had me at once update the gadgets indexed beneath with evidently derived ones. It become an entire new global for me, however I eagerly embraced those adjustments due to the fact I desired to be healed from my breast most cancers the use of extra unorthodox methods. I felt that my holistic health practitioner desired me to be healed as a whole lot as I did. My mind and emotions have been that of optimism, due to the fact I felt that if Dr Debra Williams, ND, will be healed from Stage 2 most cancers the use of herbal methods, I too will be healed!

Body Lotion
Applying lotion on your frame after a bath can assist convey a whole lot

nourishment on your pores and skin. It continues it hydrated, gentle and smooth. It is beneficial which you attempt to use lotion this is formulated in your particular pores and skin type; however, many creams may be used for more than one kinds of pores and skin.

Finding a new, all-herbal lotion for your self can also additionally once in a while be a complex process. My holistic health practitioner counseled that I use a positive kind of more virgin oil at first. I invested in it and started attempting it as a part of my each day non-public care routine. However, it reacted adversely with my pores and skin. So afterwards I become encouraged a lotion that become a stunning aggregate of tea tree oil, rice bran oil, glycerin oil, primrose oil, jojoba oil, almond oil, castor oil, avocado oil, olive oil, coconut oil and natural shea butter. This lotion now no longer simplest felt amazing, however after doing a little extra studies at the components I additionally discovered that their blessings went past simply moisturizing my pores and skin. How incredible!

I ought to be obvious with you and proportion that this lotion become extra of a economic funding that I become used to making. I become used to absolutely going to the drug shop or different splendor deliver locations and shopping for some thing I desired, or some thing become on sale. When you select to shop for all-herbal and excellent merchandise in your pores and skin, the rate factor may work up. This is only a reality of switching from a mass synthetic lotion to a excellent product. But I am extra than glad to pay extra for my health. Plus, I discovered my pores and skin to be a lot extra nurtured and more healthy searching when I switched. Truly that is the nice I even have ever used!

Deodorant

I use deodorant each day as maximum of you do as well, no doubt! It is one of these normal a part of our non-public hygiene that you can now no longer even reflect onconsideration on it. Applying your deodorant is simply as computerized as brushing your teeth. Another advice for my life-style that become made through the holistic physician become to at once put in force become to update my deodorant with a herbal one.

Now I did now no longer even understand this existed. Were most of these merchandise now no longer the

Same? Again, it got here right all the way down to the components and the way they might be dangerous to my frame. The great desire to your fitness is to pick out a deodorant that includes NO aluminum, propylene glycol or synthetic perfume. The first element to attention on is the destructive consequences of aluminum. Aluminum is located in any traditional deodorant this is labelled as an "antiperspirant." I become counseled towards the use of any deodorant with this factor because it has been connected to Alzheimer's disease, neurotoxicity (adversely affecting the imperative or peripheral apprehensive system) and breast most cancers. Considering my situation, the breast most cancers aspect piqued my hobby first, and I discovered that the aluminum will input the bloodstream via the pores and skin and through the years building up on breast tissue, that could subsequently purpose most cancers.

I become greatly surprised that this one precise factor should honestly purpose this quantity of damage withinside the frame. When I did a few extra studies on the opposite components, together with propylene glycol, I discovered that many have direct hyperlinks to acute and persistent fitness issues, along with most cancers. Again, consider the first rate adjustments that you may be developing on your frame with the aid of using surely changing one product with a obviously derived one? The herbal deodorant marketplace has definitely accelerated in current years. If you've got got buddies that use a herbal deodorant, inquire as to which manufacturers they like, or start your adventure to discover which one works for you. Look for aluminum unfastened, propylene glycol unfastened and synthetic perfume unfastened. Because each one people has distinctive frame chemistry, you could need to strive some to discover one which works for you. But going via this method is really well worth it! You are developing nice and lasting extrade on your fitness.

Toothpaste

I brush my tooth up to 3 instances a day. An marvelous reality that I discovered from my holistic physician is that the same old toothpaste you purchase from the drug or grocery keep is dangerous to your fitness! It can honestly be risky. If you examine the first-class print on toothpastes it's going to virtually state "DO NOT SWALLOW" and that if extra is swallowed than wished for brushing, you need to are looking for clinical attention. This caution by myself opened my eyes and precipitated a stir in me. It does now no longer make experience that a product that I need to installed my mouth so that you can use it may be risky in any manner if swallowed.

My holistic physician cautioned me to surely start the use of aluminum unfastened baking soda as a toothpaste. At first I concept she become joking however she become useless serious! Again, as with the whole lot there has been an adjustment. This can also additionally have felt like the largest one. Not most effective become the feel and flavor completely distinctive than what I become used to, I additionally needed to get the concept out of my head that "proper" toothpaste needed to be foamy, flavor a positive manner, and be packed with all of the chemical substances that your traditional ones are. Being as dedicated as I become, I caught with it and by no means seemed back. I am used to it now and do now no longer even consider simply the use of baking soda. It is my new normal, and I understand that if I can do it so can you! Why might you still use a product that might damage you in this type of prone location as your mouth? Even while it virtually says it may, proper at the label?

In The Home

Moving farfar from non-public care, allow us to test the following set of movement gadgets that I become requested to extrade at once so that you can start developing a more fit surroundings for my frame to heal in. Outside of private care merchandise there are numerous elements of ordinary every day exercises which you want to bear in mind of changing. The traditional manner might not be the healthiest manner. I need to percentage with you some matters that you may extrade proper now so as to prevent the cycle of harming your frame. This is all approximately now no longer bringing extra "pollution" into the home, in order that your frame can feature optimally.

Stop Using a Microwave

One of the primary adjustments I made while it got here to every day behavior withinside the kitchen become to prevent the use of a microwave altogether. When I discovered approximately the dangerous radiation that microwaves emit, I at once ceased the use of mine in my home. And later

once I moved homes, I determined now no longer to have a microwave in my new kitchen at all. There become an adjustment at first, no
Doubt. The microwave turned into brought withinside the 1950's as a high-tech addition to the kitchen, and with its evolution in layout finally have become a mainstay in kitchens everywhere in the world. People have been bought on its convenience, and in case you grew up with a microwave you won't be capable of consider your existence with out one. However, deciding on now no longer to apply a microwave, or maybe disposing of the only on your kitchen a together, is a definitive manner of preserving dangerous radiation from your home.

When I turned into suggested to forestall the use of my microwave altogether it honestly took a few being used to! No extra microwaved food or reheating matters with the pressing of a button and being capable of simply stroll away. But as I desired to enhance my fitness as exceptional I could, I commenced doing all of the cooking and reheating of meals withinside the oven or at the range top. Changing this dependancy took a piece of forethought before everything however I tailored extra fast than I expected. My buddies and own circle of relatives now additionally recognise that once they arrive to go to there may be no microwave. Funny how even for them it turned into a extrade however of path they recognise the "why" at the back of my choice and admire it fully.

Use Parchment Paper

Parchment paper has end up a staple in my kitchen after I use the oven. This is a particular form of paper that has been created to be moisture and grease resistant in addition to being capable of resist better temperatures. It is available in sheets or a roll, and may be observed withinside the segment of your grocery keep in which the wax paper or plastic wrap might also additionally be. Many humans recognise parchment as a awesome device for lining and whilst baking cookies or some thing similar. However, I now use it for everything.

In my cooking habits, parchment paper took the location of the use of any aluminum foil. As we already tested earlier, aluminum is dangerous on your body. So, I straight away switched to parchment paper and it took aluminum foil's location. I use it for cooking, baking or reheating whatever withinside the oven. It is extraordinarily smooth to apply and cleans up easily. I am surprised that it's far any other small extrade that we are able to all put into effect and one that, over time, might also additionally significantly have an effect on our fitness.

Household Cleaning Products

The third household related habit I immediately changed under the advice of my holistic practitioner was to use only all-natural cleaners in my home. Conventional cleaners that you have for things like countertops to bathrooms to floors to windows all contain harsh chemicals and compounds that essentially pollute your home. When you use them, you are introducing these chemicals into your immediate environment and exposing yourself to them. When making the switch, look for all-purpose cleaners made from plant-based ingredients which are biodegradable.

There is an intensive marketplace for herbal family cleaners. You can update each cleansing answer you've got got with one this is clearly derived. However, with a few studies I additionally observed many selfmade cleansing answers which are made with components you could have already got on your home. In fact, The Organic Consumers Association lists baking soda, borax, lemon juice, soap, Vinegar and water as "safe" cleaners. For example, I now use white vinegar as a part of some of the cleansing merchandise that I make myself. Not handiest is it inexpensive, however it has many makes use of past getting used on your cooking. Vinegar is non-poisonous and eco-friendly, making it the remaining multipurpose cleansing answer. In maximum cases, you handiest want to combine vinegar with water to create your personal all-reason cleaner. Some not unusualplace makes use of of vinegar are: appliances, tubtub tubs, counter tops, dishwashers, faucets, flooring, glass, laundry, showers, sinks and toilets. {source: Debra Rose Wilson, PhD, RN. Vinegar: The Multi-reason, Chemical-unfastened Household Cleaner You Should Know About.}

Like all modifications we were speakme about, it could take the time to conform to this new dependancy. But continually take into account the purpose you're doing it -- for the fitness of you and your cherished ones. Your cleansing merchandise do NOT should be complete of risky and vicious chemical compounds as a way to be effective.

As you still do your personal studies, I recognise you may be as amazed as I turned into at what number of makes use of there are for matters which include distinctive vinegars. Many components are so effective and multifaceted that you may be capable of assist your self in endless methods as you begin for your adventure to rid

your own home of poisonous chemical compounds. Beyond saving your fitness or even a few money, I guess you become questioning why you had now no longer been incorporating those new approaches of being a long term ago. Well, I congratulate you for being right here now, and making the modifications now. It is in no way too past due to begin a brand new bankruptcy and decide to the betterment of your fitness!

I actually have blanketed a few fundamentals with you of switching non-public care and family merchandise which might be complete of chemical compounds and toxins, to ones which might be all- herbal and secure to your fitness. Let us now consciousness in your weight loss plan. I need to have a take a observe what you're consuming, how a whole lot and when. There also are many dietary supplements that you may be taking so that you can reap foremost fitness. Again, that is all primarily based totally at the modifications that I applied in my existence that helped me remedy my breast cancer, and now sense the satisfactory I actually have in years! Let us first have a take a observe meals, and what we may be consuming to decorate our vitamins. I can't strain how critical that is.

Chapter 3

Holistic Nutrition

"The first wealth is fitness."
— **Ralph Waldo Emerson**

3

You can be acquainted with the famous saying: "You are what you devour." When it involves vitamins this could very a whole lot be taken to heart. Our our bodies will soak up the residences of the food and drink we ingest. When it comes right all the way down to it, it's miles pretty simple: in case you need to be wholesome, you should devour wholesome meals. If you need to be unhealthy, then maintain attaining for meals which might be fairly processed or unbalanced. Take a second now and replicate on what you pick out to devour. You may also in no way have virtually idea approximately it before, and in that case, I am satisfied you're right here! Maybe you try and keep away from positive matters however do now no longer be aware of the overall photograph of the whole thing you devour in a day. When it involves what you pick out to devour, you need to forestall searching at meals simply as some thing to quell your hunger. Your meals is fuel! You should extrade your attitude from meals being some thing you simply devour, to being the vitamins and vitamins you require so that you can have exquisite fitness. In the larger photograph, casting off a lot of the "consolation meals" to your weight loss plan is a small fee to pay so that you can forestall the increase and unfold of cancer.

When I become identified with breast cancer, I knew that a part of the puzzle to my healing could be converting my weight loss plan. As with the whole thing else I become converting in my existence, it become obtrusive that each element of my existence such as my nutritional selections had been affecting my fitness (and glaringly now no longer for the better). I desired to analyze what to devour so that you can optimally characteristic and to permit my frame to heal itself. If you're what you devour, I desired to be wholesome!

I SOuGht the offerings of a dietician. Together we tested what My ordinary consuming Behavior were like, after which tested my goals. Because I become seeking out meals to combat and save you cancer, they encouraged a totally unique weight loss program for me: G.B.O.M.B.S, which stands for Greens, Beans, Onions, Mushrooms, Berries, Seeds. This form of consuming plan includes complete meals, freed from some thing processed, and every meals has unique residences that could assist me in my combat in opposition to cancer. At the quit of the day though, the vitamins that this unique weight loss plan holds is exquisite for anyone!

In addition to consuming those meals I become cautioned to reduce out dairy, meat, sugar and wheat (which I simply determined difficult at first)!

I actually have many healthcare vendors in my family, so I were conscious of wholesome consuming all my existence, and up till this factor it had served me well. I felt wholesome and feature continually appeared more youthful than my real age. So a whole lot in order that I actually have even been courted via way of means of guys who had been too younger for me, due to the fact they idea I become approximately 15 years more youthful than I clearly become! But coming near a weight loss plan from this factor of view become nonetheless a shift. I become now consuming to serve my fitness, now no longer simply keep it. I become trying to create extrade in my frame and become going to apply those amazing meals as remedy in a way, now no longer simply some thing correct to devour.

I will proportion with you the unique advantages of every meals institution in my opinion, and offer a pattern listing of meals. This will come up with a few perception into expertise how every institution in my opinion can assist your frame to be nourished and running optimally to combat and save you cancer.

Greens

Green greens are the primary object at the listing of this weight loss program of holistic nutrients. My overdue mom educated as a registered nurse. Because of this, as some distance returned as I can recollect whilst we had been toddlers, our mother and father instilled in us the significance of healthful consuming. I am fortunate as I even have usually cherished greens so I had no hassle incorporating even greater into my weight loss program.

What makes inexperienced greens so suitable for you is the chlorophyll. Chlorophyll is a inexperienced pigment that facilitates greens produce and take in greater vitamins whilst going thru photosynthesis. It is taken into consideration a herbal supply of antioxidants. Antioxidants for your weight loss program are essential in stopping and combating most cancers as they defend your cells from loose radicals (which can be most cancers inflicting agents). Green greens additionally incorporate excessive quantities of magnesium and iron. Other outstanding fitness advantages except stopping most cancers include:

- Controlling blood pressure
- Strengthening your bones
- Preventing heart disease
- Improving your vision
- Boosting your immune system
- Rehydrating the body
- Aiding in weight loss
- Treating constipation
- Reducing the risk of diabetes

(Source: 10 Health Benefits of Green Vegetables via way of means of Dr. Michelle Heben)

Sample list of green vegetables:

- Artichoke
- Arugula
- Asparagus
- Bell Pepper
- Bitter Gourd
- Broccoli

- Brussels Sprouts
- Calabash
- Celery
- Chayote
- Coriander
- Cucumber
- Edamame
- Grape Leaves
- Green Beans
- Green Chili Pepper
- Green Pumpkin
- Kale
- Kohlrabi
- Leeks
- Lettuce
- Microgreens
- Okra
- Peas
- Perilla
- Ridge Gourd
- Spinach
- Watercress

- Zucchini

Beans

I even have usually understood that beans are very healthful, however I used to keep away from consuming them regularly due to the fact I could get bloated. When I lived withinside the United States, a former co-employee shared with me a mystery from his grandmother to assist save you bloating and passing wind after consuming beans. He told me to prepare dinner dinner beans with one large unpeeled Irish potato. Well, I attempted it and bingo! It labored like magic. Years later, I additionally discovered on line that setting 1 / 4 teaspoon of baking soda to 1 pound of beans will assist to save you any gaseous facet outcomes from consuming beans. This additionally labored like a charm. If you generally enjoy those type of facet outcomes from consuming beans attempt both of those techniques and I am positive they may be just right for you as well!

Also called legumes or peas, beans are seeds from the Fabaceae family. They are excessive in fiber, iron and severa vitamins. Beans also are a outstanding plant-primarily based totally protein, that's first-rate whilst seeking to reduce down or reduce out animal product consumption. Besides being a outstanding meals that contributes to most cancers prevention, additionally they have many fitness advantages that include:

- Contains folate (a type of B vitamin)
- Contains antioxidants
- Improving heart health
- Managing diabetes & glucose metabolism
- Preventing fatty liver
- Helping to control your appetite
- Improving gut health

(Source: Medical News Today)

Sample list of beans:

- Adzuki Beans
- Anasazi Beans
- Black Beans
- Black-eyed Peas
- Cannellini Beans
- Chickpeas
- Cranberry Beans
- Fava Beans
- Flageolet Beans
- Great Northern Beans
- Kidney Beans
- Lentils
- Lima Beans
- Mung Beans
- Navy Beans
- Peas
- Pinto Beans
- Red Beans
- Soybeans

Onions

One day once I became running as a hostess withinside the college membership even as pursuing my postgraduate research withinside the

United States, my pals and I had been chatting approximately one of a kind meals items. One of them delivered up the antique adage of "An apple an afternoon maintains the health practitioner away." Another co-employee shared that her grandmother used to devour a uncooked onion each day and he or she became in no way sick. Someone then exclaimed: "An onion an afternoon maintains anybody away!" Everyone laughed as onions without a doubt have and likely usually could have a recognition for his or her smelly aroma and flavor.

When it got here to growing my onion intake, I did now no longer see it as a mission at all. I without a doubt do now no longer thoughts the flavor of onions, and I became devoted to getting better.

Onions are a completely unique meals as they're cultivated and fed on throughout the globe. They are normally a temperate crop; however, they may be grown in all styles of conditions. Usually served cooked, they also can be eaten uncooked, or served in pickles or chutneys. Onions are a key meals whilst stopping or combating most cancers. A look at accomplished via way of means of the University of Guelph confirmed that purple onions had been the simplest whilst it got here to destroying breast and colon most cancers cells. This is due to the excessive ranges of quercetin and anthocyanin, compounds that immediately make contributions to this effect. Onions on an entire set off the pathways that initiate the most cancers cells to kill themselves, and create an adverse surroundings for most cancers to grow. As the most cancers cells have trouble communicating, this inhibits their growth. Some different terrific advantages of consuming onions are:

- Preventing inflammation and other allergies
- Promoting healthy digestion
- Promoting respiratory health
- Reducing oxidative stress in the body
- Lowering blood sugar levels
- Enhancing brain health
- Fights cancer... and many more!

(Source: 31 Surprising Benefits of Onions for Skin, Hair and Health via way of means of Ravi Teja Tadimalla)

Sample list of onions:

- Bermuda Onions
- Boiling Onions
- Chives
- Cipollini Onions
- Cocktail Onions
- Creole Onions
- Egyptian Onions
- Green Onions
- Leeks
- Maui Onions
- Mayan Sweet Onions
- Owa Onions
- Pearl Onions
- Pickling Onions
- Red Onions
- Red Wing Onions
- Shallots
- Spanish Onions

- Texas "Supa Sweet" Onions
- Torpedo Onions
- Tropea Lunga Onions
- Vidalia Onions
- Walla Walla Sweet Onions
- Welsh Onions
- White Onions
- Yellow Onions

Mushrooms

I used to devour mushrooms sparingly due to the fact I located them to be pretty tasteless, specially whilst eaten uncooked in salads. But I became devoted to including as a lot of them as I should into my weight loss program. I nevertheless experience they do now no longer have a whole lot flavor on their personal except they're pro very well. I even have additionally discovered the way to comprise them into outstanding recipes which might be now a part of my everyday weekly meals.

Mushroom (or toadstools) are the fleshy frame of a fungus, normally produced above ground, on soil, or on their meals supply. They may be located developing out withinside the wild, and also are cultivated and farmed. Mushrooms had been used as a supply of holistic nutrients everywhere in the global for
Centuries, because of their precise properties. Mushrooms incorporate immune helping vitamins and nutrients which could assist with shielding in opposition to numerous sorts of most cancers and retaining properly coronary heart fitness. Many of the advantages of this underrated meals organization might also additionally marvel you:

- Good source of selenium (a powerful antioxidant)
- Can help improve cholesterol

- Promotes improved gut health
- Boosts immunity
- Contain anti-inflammatory properties
- Good source of fiber
- Rich source of B vitamins
- Contain anti-cancer properties... and more!

(Source: 10 Surprising Health Benefits of Eating Mushrooms - Shalini Adams, Daily Health Body)

Sample list of mushrooms:

- Beef Steak Mushrooms
- Button Mushrooms
- Calocybe Gambosa Mushrooms
- Cauliflower Mushrooms
- Chanterelle Mushrooms
- Clamshell Mushrooms
- Cremini Mushrooms
- Enoki Mushrooms
- Hedgehog Mushrooms
- Jack-o-lantern Mushrooms
- King Oyster Mushrooms
- Lobster Mushrooms

- Maitake Mushrooms
- Meadow Mushrooms
- Milk Mushrooms
- Morel Mushrooms
- Pine Mushrooms
- Porcini Mushrooms
- Portobello Mushrooms
- Russula Mushrooms
- Shiitake Mushrooms
- St. George's Mushrooms
- White Mushrooms
- Wood Blewit Mushrooms

Berries

Eating masses of various end result has been a cornerstone of my weight loss plan for so long as I can remember. In my youngsterager years we had numerous fruit bushes at the assets wherein we lived. We loved mangoes, guavas, pineapples and others! My mom used to constantly deliver more end result to the health center wherein she labored to provide to sufferers to assist complement their diets. She might additionally inspire us to take end result to high school to percentage with friends. I am regarded to constantly have a few clean fruit in my bag, and in reality pick consuming fruit rather than simply achieving for a painkiller on the onset of a headache. I locate this easy treatment very powerful for me. For this weight loss plan I changed into requested to specially recognition on consuming berries.

Berries are small, round, juicy, pulpy, safe to eat end result. Depending at the sort of berry, they'll be discovered withinside the wild in addition to cultivated and farmed. Because in their deep and wealthy color, berries are regarded to be filled with antioxidants, which as cited earlier than are exceptional most cancers preventing agents. Cranberries specially have compounds which might be regarded to be strong most cancers preventers. Berries also are a great supply of fiber and incorporate exceptional quantities of folate (B nutrients). Other splendid advantages of berries include:

- Help manage and prevent diabetes
- Can help prevent mental decline
- All berries can help prevent heart disease
- May help prevent Alzheimer's disease
- Cranberries can prevent cancer… and more!

(Source: 15 Amazing Health Benefits of Berries with the aid of using Joseph Hindy)

Sample list of berries:

- Acai Berries
- Black Currants
- Black Raspberries
- Blackberries
- Blueberries
- Boysenberries
- Buffalo Berries
- Cape Gooseberries
- Chokeberries
- Cloudberries

- Cranberries
- Elderberries
- Goji Berries
- Golden Raspberries
- Gooseberries
- Huckleberries
- Lingonberries
- Mulberries
- Muscadine Berries
- Olalla Berries
- Pine Berries
- Red Currants
- Red Raspberries
- Salmon Berries
- Strawberries
- White Raspberries

Seeds

Seeds and nuts belong to the equal family. I sense thankful as I actually have now no longer encountered any digestive issues consuming either. Seeds are an exceptional meals. Essentially, they're embryonic vegetation which are enclosed in shielding coverings. Seeds are typically excessive in antioxidants and more healthy fat that assist in nourishing the mind and frame, that's why they may be top notch at stopping most cancers. They are a stunning entire meals and an clean addition to any weight loss plan.

Here also are a few different advantages of seeds:

- A good source of dietary fiber (which is essential for healthy digestion)
- Reduces the levels of inflammation in the body (which starves off aging reduces the risk of heart disease)
- If consumed regularly, seeds can help prevent weight loss over time

(Source: The Health Benefits of Seeds-Why You Need to Eat Them with the aid of using Nishita Kaushik)

Sample list of seeds:

- African eggplant Seeds
- Anise Seeds
- Ataiko Seeds
- Black Seeds
- Caraway Seeds
- Chia Seeds
- Coriander Seeds
- Cucumber Seeds
- Egusi Seeds
- Fennel Seeds
- Fenugreek Seeds
- Flax Seeds
- Hemp Seeds
- Iregege Seeds

- Melon Seeds
- Muskmelon Seeds
- Ogbonna Seeds
- Pine Nuts
- Pomegranate Seeds
- Poppy Seeds
- Pumpkin Seeds
- Quinoa Seeds
- Sesame Seeds
- Sunflower Seeds
- Uziza Seeds
- Watermelon Seeds
- Wild Seeds
- Yellow Mustard Seeds

Even after My BreaSt mOst cancers changed into eradicated, I saved following the G.B.O.M.B.S. weight loss plan. Not best due to the fact I am devoted to stopping any destiny cancers developing, however it additionally makes me sense complete of energy. It allows my frame sense great, and I additionally observed it allows preserve my thoughts clean as well. I recognize that for maximum of you, buying and selling for your ordinary meals for a weight loss plan of this nature can be a large change. Remember which you do now no longer should do all of it at once. You can paintings at the weight loss plan slowly however genuinely introducing greater of the required meals after which committing to creating the total overhaul.

It is only a reality of lifestyles that maximum of the time we should use dietary supplements in our diets so as to sincerely consumption a complete spectrum of nutrients and minerals. Sometimes we may want to take positive herbs for his or her particular fitness advantages. I need to percentage with you the supplementation routine that I changed into suggested to comply with for beating my breast most cancers. It is eye commencing to apprehend how particular dietary supplements in reality could make a large distinction for your standard fitness.

Chapter 4

Supplements

"I accept as true with which you can, with the aid of using taking a few easy and cheaper measures, lead an extended lifestyles and make bigger your years of well-being. My maximum essential advice is which you take nutrients each day in ultimate quantities to complement the nutrients which you acquire for your meals."
— Linus Pauling

Food dietary supplements are focused reassets of vitamins (nutrients and minerals) or different herbs which have particular physiological and mental outcomes at the frame. Each complement has a encouraged dose that it's miles administered in, and need to be accompanied cautiously as there may be this kind of component as "an excessive amount of of a great component." All dietary supplements may be discovered over-the-counter at your nearby pharmacy or fitness meals store. They aren't regulated with the aid of using americaA Food and Drug Administration, so it's miles vital which you purchase your dietary supplements from relied on and respectable brands.

Taking your nutrients can cross to this point past simply popping a multivitamin and being accomplished for the day. It may be visible as every other manner to aid your frame and all its systems, so you can lead an optimally wholesome existence. Based at the kingdom of my failing fitness after I started preventing my most cancers, of direction I became up for including any and all dietary supplements to my diet. I sincerely nearly predicted to, as I already understood how effective they may be. My holistic practitioner strongly suggested me to observe a listing of each day dietary supplements so as to enhance my immune gadget. Again, those encouraged dietary supplements have been particular to what I became attempting to perform fitness-wise.

YOu can Be thinking why, if I becaMe following a Strict G.B.O.M.B.S. diet, I might want extra dietary supplements. Supplements could make up for the reality that a few vitamins are misplaced while you prepare dinner dinner your meals. Also, it's far very beneficial in case you can not devour all of your meals from natural reassets as a few end result and veggies can be sprayed with preservatives for transportation to the grocery store. I continually attempt to shop for all my sparkling produce from the farmers marketplace withinside the summer, so I am taking the hottest and maximum to be had supply of vitamins that I can. Here are a few different very vital motives why a few human beings can also additionally take dietary supplements:

- Filling in any nutritional gaps (based on food availability or poor e habits)
- Nutrient absorption declines with age
- Regular exercise can increase nutrient needs
- Depletion of nutrients in the soil

- Preventative measures to more expensive health issues down the road

(Source: Whole Health for the reason that 1997, December 16, 2020)

You are greater than welcome to attempt any and all dietary supplements. Most may be secure so long as you observe the guidelines indexed at the label. However, in case you are new to the usage of dietary supplements, I propose which you visit a herbal physician earlier than starting.

Vitamin B

Taking a Vitamin B complicated became the primary at the listing of dietary supplements to contain into my each day routine. A Vitamin B complicated is a particular combination of B nutrients this is dosed especially to every one, however altogether in a single capsule. You see, every B nutrition has distinctive houses with a purpose to have an effect on the frame differently. Perhaps you probably did now no longer understand that there are multiple B nutrition? Yes, there are! A photograph of a B nutrition complicated will include:

- B-1 (thiamine)
- B-2 (riboflavin)
- B-3 (niacin)
- B-5 (pantothenic acid)
- B-6 (pyridoxine)
- B-7 (biotin)
- B-9 (folic acid)
- B-12 (cobalamin)

As I mentioned, every B nutrition can play a completely particular position withinside the frame. For my purposes, I became taking it for my mobileular fitness and immune gadget. Other approaches that B nutrition complicated can also additionally have an effect on your basic fitness are:

- Improving energy levels
- Stimulating growth of red blood cells
- Encouraging healthy brain function
- Assisting your cardiovascular health
- and more!

(Source: Health Line)

Vitamin C

Vitamin C is likewise called ascorbic acid and ascorbate. It is ample in lots of foods, however additionally provided as a nutritional supplement. Vitamin C is an crucial nutrient with regards to repairing tissues on your frame, and is needed for the functioning of numerous enzymes. It is likewise called one of the crucial vitamins to your immune gadget fitness.

Other advantages of Vitamin C include:

- Improving mood and mental health
- Acting as an antioxidant, fights oxidative damage.
- Supporting and regenerating Vitamin E
- Increasing calcium absorption (in turn assisting with bone health)
- Enhancing the absorption of nonheme iron
- It may help to reduce the risk of cardiovascular disease

(Source: Nutrition advance, 2021)

Vitamin D3 +K2 + A

You can also additionally have heard of the advantages of Vitamin D3, mainly in case you stay withinside the northern hemisphere. D3 is continuously spoken approximately due to its recognition for being the "solar nutrition." Essentially the handiest herbal supply of Vitamin D3 is the real solar being absorbed through your skin, in any other case you ought to take a supplement! Vitamin D3 is fundamental to many frame capabilities which includes constructing your immune gadget. However, it's far now recognised that after you are taking D3, it's far most useful to take it with a K2. The motive at the back of that is that each want to be mixed so as for the D3 to be comfortably absorbed through your frame.

When referring especially to breast most cancers, a take a look at offered withinside the "American Journal of Epidemiology" (through Dr. Eric Horlick) observed that after a person became uncovered to greater solar and had ok nutrition D manufacturing of their younger person years, their danger for breast most cancers later in person existence extensively decreased. Further studies cautioned that enough stages of Vitamin D may additionally lessen the danger of colorectal, prostate and pancreatic most cancers, to call a few. In one take a look at of 34,000 adults, people with excessive stages of Vitamin D had a 20 percentage decrease threat of growing all kinds of most cancers. How incredible!

Some different advantages of Vitamin D include:

- Healthier pregnancies for moms and babies
- Wards off autoimmune disease
- Helps prevent colds and the flu
- Improves all aspects of heart health
- Boosts your mood
- Eases IBS (irritable bowel syndrome); abdominal pain, bloating, diar and constipation
- Helps protect against autism
- Increases general life expectancy
- and more!

(Source: Denise Mann- Best Health)

Vitamin E

Taking Vitamin E every day is some other manner to complement your weight loss program to encompass extra most cancers preventing power. Vitamin E is a effective antioxidant, which as I cited earlier than is a key element in preventing unfastened radicals withinside the body. Antioxidant houses shield your cells and DNA from harm that unfastened radicals or most cancers cells can cause. Vitamin E is crucial in relation to assisting your vision, reproductive fitness and the general fitness of your blood, mind and skin.

Some different advantages can also additionally encompass:

- Fades scars and stretch marks
- Fights wrinkles
- Protects you from sun damage
- Reduces the risk of heart disease
- Fights osteoarthritis inflammation
- Boosts your immune system
- and more!

(Source: Dr. Michelle Heben, drhealthbenefit.com)

Moringa Oleifera Capsules

Moringa Oleifera is maximum normally called Moringa. It is a plant this is local to northern India. You can also additionally have additionally heard it called drumstick tree, horseradish tree or maybe ben oil tree. It comes to be had as a powder that you may have as a tea or on your smoothies, or as capsules. Moringa turned into advocated to be a part of my weight loss program for its anti-most cancers effects. This is due to the fact it's far filled with antioxidants which as we now understand increase the immune machine and shield cells from unfastened radical harm.

Other advantages of the usage of Moringa encompass:

- A potent source of vitamin C (about 7 times the amount of vitamin C would get from eating an orange!)
- Provides 3 times the amount of iron than in a cup of spinach
- Provides 4 times the amount of vitamin A than from one carrot
- Includes potassium, calcium, and protein!
- Includes amino acids that support the immune system

(Source: Ken Wiginton medically reviewed via way of means of Melinda Ratini, DO, MS)

Red Reishi Micronized Mushroom Capsules

Remember withinside the remaining bankruptcy after I cited the way it turned into advocated to start consuming mushrooms as one of the fundamental meals organizations of my new weight loss program? Well, right here we're and certainly considered one among my dietary supplements that turned into advocated to me is likewise a mushroom! My holistic practitioner by no means ceases to amaze me together along with her exclusive protocols. I commenced taking Red Reishi mushrooms that were dried and dosed especially into capsules.

Many humans frequently devour this mushroom for its capability most cancers preventing houses. A look at that protected 4000 breast most cancers survivors located that 59% frequently fed on Reishi mushrooms. Other advantages of this top notch meals encompass:

- Boosting the immune system
- Fighting fatigue and depression
- Improving heart health
- Controlling blood sugar

- Having high antioxidant status

(Source: Healthline.com)

As you may see, the significance of supplementing your weight loss program in exclusive methods may be especially beneficial, specially whilst handling precise fitness problems which include preventing or stopping most cancers. Engaging with a holistic practitioner and developing your personal supplementation routine can be the price price tag to feeling in higher fitness, now and withinside the future.

I even have shared the primary steps I took whilst overhauling my weight loss program. I recall after I took on the overall meals and supplementation plan as directed, and I felt great. I recall feeling nourished and stimulated as I knew I turned into including some other layer of care to my everyday combat in opposition to my breast most cancers. The 1/3 a part of my weight loss program overhaul turned into now equipped to be introduced. I turned into now no longer acquainted with intermittent fasting earlier than my holistic practitioner delivered it to my interest to consider. Now I can't consider now no longer following those hints to consuming! Keep an open thoughts and allow us to dive into the following a part of our journey.

Chapter 5

Intermittent Fasting

> *"Fasting or intermittent fasting offers us an possibility to certainly get all of the quality cells all of the time and that's what all of us want."*
> — Dr. Steven Gundry

5

I turned into so excited at this factor on my most cancers preventing journey. At this factor my existence turned into starting to appearance considerably exclusive in phrases of the alternatives I turned into making for my surroundings and my weight loss program. I had one extra shift to make though, whilst it got here to my weight loss program, and it turned into now no longer approximately what I turned into consuming, it needed to do with after I turned into selecting to eat. My holistic practitioner advocated me to attempt intermittent fasting in my new lifestyle. I turned into hesitant. I had heard of this practice, however some thing to do with fasting appeared like a huge undertaking. The most effective fasting I turned into acquainted with turned into certainly in a extra spiritual context and now no longer a part of a everyday lifestyle. But as with the whole thing else my holistic practitioner turned into suggesting, I turned into extra than inclined to tackle any and all adjustments that might help in assisting me combat my breast most cancers.

I had attempted fasting earlier than, so the concept of it became now no longer a hundred percent new to me. Of course, after I first attempted fasting, it became a challenge. But in the end you do get used to it! As a part of our practices at church, we'd often speedy as a congregation. Due to a few preexisting scientific situations I became dealing with, I became allowed to devour end result which took "the edge" off, as a way to speak. I additionally needed to remember as I have been dealing with anemia as nicely throughout a few instances of fasting. That became all below manage earlier than I commenced intermittent fasting as a part of my regime to overcome breast cancer. However, as we on occasion do now no longer realize a hundred percent what goes on in our bodies, it's miles continually excellent to test in together along with your medical doctor or different medical doctor as a way to make certain you may be installation for success.

What is Fasting?

Fasting goes with none meals or drink for a particular quantity of time. Fasting has generally been referred to as a part of spiritual practices or additionally engaged in for non-public reasons. During a quick clearly no meals is taken,
and commonly no drinks either (and which can additionally encompass water).

Fasting is definitely now no longer for everyone. For example, pregnant ladies and people with positive pre-current scientific situations are cautioned now no longer to speedy. If you're thinking about project any type of fasting protocol, please are seeking for scientific recommendation first.

Different Types of Fasting

There are many forms of fasting that every one serve exceptional purposes. I need to spotlight some so you can also additionally then have the ability to differentiate them a chunk higher. Not simplest for yourself, however additionally to have higher knowledge and be supportive of every person you can come upon who's fasting.

Absolute speedy: Another call for this is "dry fasting." This fasting does now no longer permit any water intake, in conjunction with the standard abstaining from all meals and different drink.

Partial speedy: This can seek advice from omitting one meal a day. Or it could seem like simplest consuming positive end result and veggies for numerous days at a time.

Rotational speedy: Certain ingredients are averted periodically. For example, grains aren't eaten for numerous days then protected withinside the food plan for numerous days.

Liquid speedy: Abstaining from stable meals however bearing in mind all fluids (juices, milks, tea, water).

People have interaction in fasting for lots exceptional reasons. Fasts are linked to spiritual vacations for lots exceptional religions. They can also additionally characterize acknowledging a specific tale the vacation is targeted around, or function a manner to connect with the Divine or God. Fasting is significantly related to a time for deep internal contemplation, and to function a manner of higher knowledge oneself.

For my precise desires my holistic practitioner helped educate me approximately intermittent fasting and the way it could be part of my restoration journey.

Why Intermittent Fasting?

You can also additionally have heard of intermittent fasting already, because it has won reputation in current years. As mentioned, the center concept is which you limition all consuming and consuming to simplest a specific term of your day. This allows you derive a number of the advantages of fasting, while not having to head with out meals for an prolonged duration of time. There are many bureaucracy that you could select (in phrases of the time intervals); however, "sixteen/eight" is the maximum famous. sixteen/eight is used to suggest which you speedy for sixteen hours after which are approved to devour in the eight-hour window of time in keeping with people's schedules. Many select to devour among the hours of 12 midday and 8pm.

Benefits of Intermittent Fasting

The sixteen/eight intermittent fasting version is a famous food plan because it is simple to follow, bendy and feels sustainable lengthy term. Depending on what goes on for your time table possibly you turn your hours to a bit in advance or a bit later. What truely counts is sticking to sixteen hours of fasting throughout a 24- hour cycle. In phrases of affecting your fitness, sixteen/eight intermittent fasting has been related to many fitness advantages that encompass:

Increased weight loss: Because of the shorter window for consuming, you'll obviously reduce energy as you're clearly consuming less. Studies have additionally proven that fasting for a part of the day can also additionally boom metabolism and consequently assist with weight loss.

Improved blood sugar manage: Studies have observed whilst often practising intermittent fasting, fasting insulin ranges were decreased as much as 31% and decrease your blood sugar with the aid of using 3-6% (all in all of your standard threat of diabetes).

Longer and all-spherical more healthy lifestyles: A latest observe with the aid of using Harvard researchers confirmed that fasting altered the mitochondrial hobby in our cells. (Mitochondria are answerable for changing meals into strength that the mobileular can use.) This can also additionally growth lifespan, sluggish the fee of getting old and enhance typical health. (Source: Fasting: The Forgotten Cure with the aid of using Josephine Marcellin)

Different Types of Intermittent Fasting

It is crucial to renowned that withinside the realm of intermittent fasting there are numerous routes you may take. I will define them for you, However maintain in thoughts that for my functions of looking to be cancer-unfastened and save you destiny cancer, I became advocated to particularly comply with the 16/eight method. However, I need to offer you with as lots statistics that I can so you can also additionally preserve to do your personal investigations as to what can be proper for you, relying to your health.

16/eight Method: This shows the sample for limiting all meals consumption to handiest an eight-hour window of 24 hrs. Beyond which you are allowed water, black espresso or tea, and another 0 energy beverages.

five/2 Diet: In this healthy dietweight-reduction plan you devour generally for five days of your week and throughout the alternative 2 days you limition your energy. It is usually recommended 500 energy for girls and six hundred energy for guys at the 2 "fasting" days.

"Eat. Stop. Eat." Method: This entails a complete speedy for twenty-four hours a couple of times a week. An instance of what this can appear to be is to prevent consuming after dinner at 7pm, then to now no longer devour till 7pm the subsequent day. Whatever agenda works for you.

Alternate Day Fasting: This is committing to fasting each different day both with the aid of using absolutely now no longer consuming or handiest consuming some hundred energy to maintain you.

Warrior Diet: This eating regimen seems like consuming a minimum quantity of entire end result and veggies throughout the day then consuming one massive balanced meal at night time. So basically you're in a semi speedy maximum of the day then destroy it at night time with dinner.

(Source: Healthline.com/nutrition/6-ways-to-do-intermittent fasting)

My Personal Journey with Intermittent Fasting

As I referred to earlier, I already had a records with fasting thru my church on the time. So, undertaking intermittent fasting got here plenty simpler than I had expected. I nonetheless exercise my 16/eight intermittent fasting, however handiest Monday thru Friday. Now that it's miles simply a part of my preservation plan, I permit no time regulations on my consuming throughout the weekend, and locate that makes it plenty simpler whilst socializing with pals or commercial enterprise partners.

During my adventure with intermittent fasting, I observed many high-quality adjustments with my body:

- I lost 10 pounds without focusing on that. The weight just came off.
- My body became more agile and flexible.
- I no longer experience pain in my joints.
- I no longer experience bloating as I had prior to practicing intermi fasting.
- I am able to ingest more liquids, so staying hydrated no longer feels l challenge.
- I have more energy! So much in fact that I am able to go for walk 30 min every morning AND then do another 30 minutes of aerobic exercise w get home.
- I look and feel younger!

During a zoom convention I became tuning into, a celeb athlete stated:

"Many of you fall unwell due to the fact you devour too frequently." This genuinely piqued my hobby as that gave the impression of a model of fasting to me. When I referred to this assertion to my holistic practitioner, she added: "And humans additionally fall unwell due to the fact they devour an excessive amount of meals." Dr. Miriam Merad, lead writer of a brand new fasting observe, stated food an afternoon can be perfect for human health. (Source: Hilary Brueck.) Reflecting by myself studies and private revel in it's miles very clean to me that intermittent fasting (and different kinds of fasting) have a particular and crucial position to play in our typical health.

In the closing 3 chapters we've mentioned the whole thing to do with meals: what to devour, whilst to devour, and the way to complement your eating regimen. I wish you sense like you've got got a stable leaping off factor to discover those components of recovery for your self.

As motivational speaker Zig Ziglar stated, "If you assist sufficient humans get what they need, you may get what you need." I am searching ahead to now leaping into speaking approximately concerning your self withinside the network as a manner to additionally heal and save you disease.

Chapter 6

Plant Good Seeds

"We make a residing with the aid of

using what we get, however we make a lifestyles with the aid of using what we provide."
— Winston Churchill

6

Part of my lifestyles that I desired to recognition on whilst I became in my recovery adventure became giving lower back: now no longer handiest to my network however to the arena as a entire. When you provide to others you boost the coolest strength on your lifestyles. Giving lower back and contributing to the arena is acknowledging which you are a part of a larger picture. Your lifestyles does now no longer simply consist of your work, own circle of relatives and pals. We are all a part of a larger network, be it regionally or globally.

When I commenced my restoration adventure, this have become very obvious to me. Even aleven though I become going via a hard time, I ought to nonetheless take time to provide returned. Taking consciousness farfar from my personal demanding situations for some time and assisting elevate a person else up become a vital aspect of my restoration. Sometimes those have been movements I become already engaged in. Sometimes I determined new approaches to get involved. Either manner it did now no longer matter, it stays an critical a part of my weekly schedule.

I will percentage with you a few approaches that I deliver returned or "plant proper seeds." This is all in desire which you are then capable of study your personal existence and approaches that you could deliver returned in case you aren't already, or remain stimulated to make contributions to the network round you. Giving returned fills your existence on an entire with more that means and purpose... No surprise it become such an critical a part of my restoration adventure and is still a focal point of mine. There are many wonderful approaches to make contributions. Let us begin with one of the maximum famous and simplest approaches to provide returned, with the aid of using supplying your time.

Volunteering

Volunteering your time, strength and capabilities to a purpose is such an tremendous manner to have interaction together along with your existence. Through volunteering you without delay deliver returned to the network. At the equal time, you'll maximum truely meet many varieties of human beings with exceptional capabilities and talents. Taking the time to volunteer can show to be such an powerful manner of increasing your self as a person.

Volunteering commonly entails placing your self in new situations. With that comes the opportunity of now no longer simplest gaining new capabilities, however additionally enhancing your self-esteem. Taking day trip of your personal existence to advantage the lives of others makes you experience humble and complete of gratitude. Volunteering has been determined to certainly growth your existence expectancy! (source:breakingnewsenglish.com). I experience the reasoning in the back of that is clear. When you experience beneficial and a part of some thing larger than your self, your strength shifts to vibrate higher. It isn't always a accident that your fitness could be bolstered.

Also, folks who deliver, entice proper matters into their lives! Maybe you've got got skilled this your self. Or possibly you realize a person who continually appears to draw remarkable matters into their lives, be it cloth or otherwise. It is virtually how the sector works. If you deliver proper matters, proper matters will come returned to you.

You can are searching for out volunteer possibilities or you could even create your personal. Get innovative and continually make contributions in a manner that feels aligned with you. To lend a few inspiration, permit me percentage with you my enjoy of the way I got here to sign up for a crew of folks who consciousness on feeding impoverished participants of my network.

My Experience of Giving Back

When I offered my new apartmentminium in October 2020, my actual property agent counseled that earlier than I moved into the space, I ask a pastor to return back with the aid of using and bless this new domestic for me. I cherished this idea! I positioned the phrase out, and a chum delivered me to a pastor who blesses houses as a part of his job. The pastor arrived

together along with his spouse and the pal we had in common. After an hour of blessing my apartmentminium, reciting scriptures, analyzing from the Bible, taking in a mini sermon from the pastor, in addition to blessing my apartmentminium with greater virgin oil and water, his spouse requested me if I would love to accompany them to feed the homeless. They installation a desk as soon as every week in one of the slums in
downtown Toronto in which they provided a warm meal to every body who wished one. I wholeheartedly agreed! I couldn't assist however replicate on pix of former President Barack Obama, First Lady Michelle Obama and their own circle of relatives assisting serve at a soup kitchen on Thanksgiving Day... I felt aligned with giving returned on this manner.

Spearheaded with the aid of using the pastor, each Sunday we installation a desk at the sidewalk and commit time to provide a nutritious, balanced meal in addition to water and juice. We additionally provide face mask and hand sanitizers to take for non-public use. One week, we observed every other institution of human beings withinside the location of our desk dispensing sandwiches. It become tremendous that every other institution become additionally organizing and giving returned to the ones in want in our network.

It is simply too clean to take existence for granted! After donating my time to feeding the ones in my network who've much less than me, I am endlessly thankful to The Almighty for the reality that I actually have food, refuge and clothing. I not take whatever for granted, and experience blessed for all I actually have and all this is coming my manner. I love donating my time to this purpose.

Donating to Charitable Causes

There are hundreds of thousands of charities installation all around the world, with the aim to elevate cash for the ones in want. A charity can be huge and goal a bigger hassle or populace of people. However, now and again they may be very small and specialized. There are a whole lot of blessings of donating to a charity, from the overall to personal:

- Inspire and create civic engagement (which is so important to build h communities)

- Elevate your community standing
- Reduce your rates of stress and feel more satisfied with your life in gene
- Feel more joy!
- Activate the reward center in your brain

(Source: Mary McCoy, certified Social Worker)

    I determined that I desired to start creating a ordinary donation to a charity that I felt aligned with. I did a few studies and on the stop of the day I determined to decide to donating to The Mary Kay Ash Charitable Foundation each month. The Mary Kay Ash Charitable Foundation allows keep on Mary Kay's legacy with its unified task to aid ladies residing with most cancers and to place an stop to home violence. (Source: About Mary Kay-Our History). I become aware about the charity as I am a former impartial Mary Kay Beauty Consultant. However, due to the fact I am an authorized network French interpreter and now a breast most cancers survivor, this charity now aligns with my very own dreams and vision.

    The Mary Kay Ash Charitable Foundation takes 1/2 of their donations and gives investment to aid studies especially centered at casting off cancers that without delay have an effect on ladies. Now as a breast most cancers survivor, I need with the intention to provide returned to the opportunity of assisting different ladies who do now no longer should undergo this revel in withinside the future. The different 1/2 of in their charitable version is in attempt to stop the epidemic of home violence in opposition to ladies via supplying presents that help network outreach packages in addition to ladies's shelters. As an authorized network French interpreter, I paintings in lots of extraordinary settings which encompass social services. I had been known as to offer interpretation in extraordinary conditions at numerous ladies's shelters, the Children's Aid Society, police stations, detention centers, hospitals and different inclined places. I even have heard firsthand the awful memories of home violence and abuse that ladies have needed to endure. I need to make contributions to assist stop this cycle of violence in opposition to ladies.

    As you could see, I discovered a charity that virtually aligns with my existence and values. If you do now no longer have already got a charity which you realize of which you already aid or would really like to, begin

doing a little studies. I am certain that there are a few reasons which you both in my view align with, or that talk without delay in your values. Find a charity which you love and couldn't imagine
NOT giving your cash to. Remember, for lots charities each unmarried greenback counts, so even in case your donation is pretty humble it's far really well worth a lot. Do what you could with what you have. It is all a part of planting suitable seeds.

Supporting Each Other

We have tested approaches you could provide returned to the outer circles on your existence. What approximately giving returned in your greater internal and private circles? What approximately giving returned to folks that can be a part of your existence already, however do now no longer always want economic assistance? Perhaps there are possibilities on your existence wherein you could provide returned via your time, presence and ideas. This can seem like being a part of a network organization or possibly even via a greater expert improvement lens. I am fortunate as I even have numerous approaches in my existence that I am capable of make contributions to extraordinary circles or people's lives the use of now no longer best my time, however additionally via using abilities I even have evolved over the years. I would like to proportion greater with you in hopes of inspiring you to comprehend extraordinary approaches that you will be capable of provide returned to connections which might be already mounted on your existence.

Remember the pastor who ran the outreach initiative to feed underserviced participants of my network? Well, he runs a Bible take a look at organization that I am so thankful to be a element of. As the call suggests, a Bible take a look at organization is a set of folks who often get collectively to take a look at the phrase of God, be it thru analyzing the Bible, preaching or reciting intercessory prayers. My organization meets each day for half-hour withinside the early morning, and we behavior our organization over the smartphone as our participants live in each Canada and withinside the United States. We all make a contribution with the aid of using announcing prayers or readings on a rotating basis. The pastor stocks a sermon and continually activates us with matters to mirror upon. Gathering in a Bible take a look at organization can provide such a lot of possibilities to connect with matters which are extra than you, and may be an area of boom and healing. I actually have had my very own non-public breakthroughs, all of the even as making new pals and assisting them and their breakthroughs. It is a unique and intimate circle of like-minded human beings that I actually have great gratitude for.

Another manner I plant precise seeds in my lifestyles is with the aid of using being a member of a mastermind alliance. These styles of organizations have existed considering that time immemorial! However, it turned into Napoleon Hill who described a mastermind alliance and its capability withinside the ee-e book Think and Grow Rich in 1937. Since then, organizations all around the international have fashioned with the goal of accumulating in a based surroundings and sharing in every other's wins and losses. My mastermind meets each Saturday morning for 2 hours. During that time, we every have an possibility to proportion and dissect the advances or setbacks of our goals. We alternate thoughts and outdoor views for non-public development. Each folks has our very own strengths and knowledge that we will carry to the organization. That is why those organizations are notably unique and critical. Our organization is known as the Eagles mastermind alliance and there's no funding to join. We have studied the ee-e book Think and Grow Rich and are presently analyzing The Law of Success in Sixteen Lessons. Both books had been written with the aid of using Napoleon Hill. We are devoted to every other's achievement and assisting each other as we try for excellence. Not simplest have I located human beings to collaborate with on thrilling thoughts, I actually have additionally made lasting friendships.

In my professional life, I am very proud to have acquired three coaching designations. I received my Distinguished Toastmasters designation (the highest accolade bestowed on a Toastmasters member, obtained by only two percent of Toastmasters) through which I went on to mentor Toastmasters members. After obtaining my Distinguished Toastmasters designation, I ventured out and obtained a World Class Speaking Coach certificate from Craig Valentine, MBA (1999 World Class champion of Toastmasters). Toastmasters International is a worldwide non-profit educational organization that empowers individuals to become more effective communicators and leaders. Headquartered in Englewood, Colorado, USA, the organization's membership exceeds 357,000 people in more than 16,600 clubs in 143 countries. {Source: https://www.toastmasters.org}

Furthermore, I have become a licensed instruct, speaker and teacher thru The John Maxwell Company, which noticed me being capable of practice competencies discovered to be able to educate French to global college students on a non-public platform.

Currently, I am additionally enrolled in a direction to emerge as a licensed fitness and lifestyles instruct with the intention to be licensed in 2022. I love being capable of assist human beings stage up their very own competencies to be able to discover new stages of achievement, irrespective of what they may be seeking to achieve. It seems like such an critical issue of why I am here. You may even see this thru my penning this ee-e book! I need to peer human beings be triumphant and thrive, and need to assist in any manner I can. I need to plant any precise seeds, massive or small, round me in order that I might also additionally watch a lovely lawn of capability boom.

Of direction, being of carrier to the ones round you in distinct approaches is of top notch importance. However, you may in no way overlook to additionally display up for yourself. You can not simply positioned your very own wellbeing at the lower back burner and desire that you'll be OK. You ought to learn how to make investments time and power into your very own self-care as well, so you can preserve displaying up to your pals, own circle of relatives and network time and time again. Self-care wishes to be a concern to your lifestyles. No excuses!

Chapter 7

Self-Care

> *"I deal with myself quite precise. I take plenty of vacation, I devour well, I take supplements, I do mercury detox,*
> *I get masses of sleep. I drink masses of water and I live farfar from drama and stress."*
> — Reba McEntire

7

Self-care can imply various things for one of a kind human beings. When it comes right all the way down to it, it does now no longer rely what it truly appears like, however adopting amazing self-care practices is sincerely important whilst trying to beat most cancers or assist save you it. Everything we've got mentioned thus far may be notion of as your basis. The weight loss program and the whole thing we've got spoken of include non-negotiables. Now upon that basis you need to construct a self-care ordinary for your self.

Perhaps you have already got a self-care ordinary that you could simply start to contain as soon as your basis is in place. Fantastic! Start from there and additionally be open to new ideas. If constructing a self-care ordinary is new to you, do now no longer worry. You can start with the aid of using exploring what feels proper for you. Maybe there are already a few matters that pique your hobby which you have constantly desired to try. Or possibly you don't have any concept wherein to start.

I will percentage with you a few practices that I recollect a part of my selfcare ordinary. Feel loose to apply them as leaping off factors in your personal exploration. Do now no longer forget, self-care need to experience proper. It need to now no longer experience like a chore, or some thing you need to presSure your self thru. Sure, you can must contain a few area to reveal as much as what you want to do. However, self-care need to truely experience just like the icing at the cake in relation to including to the ordinary you're already cultivating.

Exercise Regimen

I actually have constantly had a few kind of exercising regime. Exercise makes me experience calm, healthful and relaxed. It additionally makes me sleep better. Because my mom became a registered nurse, from an early age each my mother and father constantly instilled in us the significance of exercising. I recall driving a bicycle from formative years into my teenage years, or even loving hiking the fruit trees
that had been in our backyard. My siblings and I extensively utilized to revel in going swimming regularly. Being energetic became a herbal a part of my every day lifestyles. My mom constantly used to say: "If you need to stay long, exercising!" She is a testomony of this declaration due to the fact she went for walks till the ripe age of 85!

Prior to the Covid-19 pandemic, I participated in swimming and aquafit classes. (If you aren't acquainted with aquafit, it's miles wherein you basically do aerobics in a swimming pool. It may be very amusing!) However, due to pandemic guidelines the swimming pool closed in my apartmentminium and I needed to discover different approaches to hold fit. Fitness had emerge as such part of my lifestyles that I had to adapt which will ensure it stayed a part of my ordinary.

I determined to tackle aerobics and brisk on foot due to the fact they had been cost- powerful and amusing to do. Aerobics can provide you a lot with such little time commitment:

- Improves the efficiency of respiration
- Improves cardiovascular efficiency
- Strengthens your muscles
- Strengthens ligaments, tendons and bones
- Helps decrease anxiety and stress
- Helps decrease the risk of developing cancer, coronary artery dis diabetes ... and more!

(Source: Ask an Expert: The Benefits of Aerobic Exercise. Providence Health

& Services Oregon and Southwest Washington)

The blessings of exercising as a part of a healthful manner of residing has been documented time and time again. However, in case you are present process most cancers remedy of any sort, it's miles particularly vital. The blessings are substantial and might include:

- Reducing the onset of anxiety and depression

- Lowering the chance of having physical side effects such as fat lymphedema (when legs and arms swell due to fluid retention), neurop (damage or dysfunction of nerves), osteoporosis and nausea

- Helping you remain as physically independent and mobile as possible

- Improving sleep. It is so important to get good sleep all the time especially when undergoing treatment as it provides a chance for your to heal.

- Helping reduce the risks of other cancers, and can act as prevent medicine

- It improves the survival rates for certain cancers such as breast and rectal cancers

- and many more!

(Source: most cancers.net/survivorship/healthful-residing/erxercise-during-most cancers- remedy)

Having an exercising routine will enhance your pleasant of lifestyles regardless of what goes on. This is why it could be visible as an vital a part of your self- care ordinary. It can't handiest assist you experience proper withinside the moment, however is such an asset in your destiny health. Many human beings exercising now no longer due to how they need to experience today, however due to how they need to experience withinside the days and the years to come! Find what works for you. It does now no longer must be a main commitment. The rule of thumb is to sweat approximately 20 mins a day. Find what sports get you transferring and discover what time of day you experience great fits you. Perhaps you do some thing first factor withinside the morning and use it as an power booster. Or possibly you exercising withinside the afternoon as a select out me up. Explore and get creative. Create your personal dating to transferring your frame and this shape of self-care.

Breast Care

When I had the tumuor in my proper breast removed, the oncologist became so compassionate that he even apologized for leaving scars from the surgery. I advised him that it became okay, due to the fact lifestyles is complete of scars. As I actually have found out thru this journey, our scars grow to be stars, our shame into grace and our mess right into a message.

My oncologist encouraged I put on a snug sports activities bra for 6 weeks after my surgery. He encouraged a sports activities bra in particular due to the fact they do now no longer have any underwire constructed into them. I later determined out from a pal of mine who's a nurse that underwire bras may Also motive breast most cancers with the aid of using blocking off the drainage of lymph fluid from the lowest of the breast so it can not get returned into your body. Also, I quick located that sports activities bras are extra snug than traditional ones (specially while improving from surgery). After the six weeks I persevered to put on sports activities bras as an awful lot as viable as I determined them extraordinarily snug.

I discover it exciting as the problem of sporting bras became added up additionally with the homeopathic health practitioner I cited I had visible in 2014. After diagnosing that my proper breast had now no longer been functioning nicely, the homeopathic health practitioner cautioned that I need to now no longer put on a bra at home, or every time I did now no longer have to. I even have taken all of this recommendation to coronary heart. I not put on a bra, as an awful lot as viable. I am very aware of this, as I now apprehend that it isn't a terrific concept for my breast fitness. While bras are part of life, it has end up very clean to me that it isn't wholesome for the breasts themselves to usually be sporting a bra. If you're a woman, I need you to take that to coronary heart and forestall sporting your bra as an awful lot as you may. Or possibly put on a sports activities bra extra as they're much less restrictive for the tissues. I do not forget as a teenager, while my mom lower back home, she could usually dispose of her bra... now I apprehend why!

There is an old concept that sporting a bra is notion to help the

improvement of organization and nicely-fashioned breasts. However, new findings are proving this isn't true. Studies were constantly displaying that bras do now no longer save you sagging or enhance breast fitness in any manner. They may also
without a doubt be pretty unfavorable to the general appearance of the breast and extra importantly be unfavorable in generating wholesome breast tissue.

(Source: Benefits of going braless-Breast Enlargement Resource)

In phrases of different ways, you may control the fitness of your breast tissue is to without a doubt supply your breasts a rubdown often. There are a few Registered Massage Therapists who provide breast rubdown. However, you may additionally do it yourself. I often rubdown my breasts, specially after the bathe after I am making use of moisturizer to my body. It is an extremely good brief and clean manner to feature in your every day self-care. I these days discovered from a registered nurse that the right manner to rubdown breasts is to rub every breast fifty instances each clockwise and anticlockwise to permit blood to flow into freely. I do not forget after I met with a homeopathic health practitioner, he additionally cautioned me to rubdown my breast in a comparable fashion.

As a part of my normal put up most cancers care, I even have annual mammograms and ultrasounds on each my breasts. While that is vital for me thinking about my fitness history, I suggest speakme in your fitness care company approximately normal mammograms. This is an extremely good a part of preventative medicine. Part of the fulfillment of most cancers prognosis is early detection, and one manner to come across a lump is while having a mammogram. I had in advance cited that mammograms aren't hundred percentage accurate. I stuck the lump in my breast via self-examination. Because of my very own ultrasounds, my oncologist became absolutely capable of advantage perception as to how nicely my opportunity remedies have been working, and maintain to hold my breasts most cancers-free. It is vital to get a feel of your breast fitness from the inner out with the intention to speak.

I will reiterate the significance of breast self-examinations because the first-class manner to discover a lump while it's far in its infancy. Again, in case you are uncomfortable touching your very own breasts, ask your associate to do it. If you do now no longer have a associate, be inclined to pay a rubdown therapist to do it for you. Incorporating this into your recurring may also shop your life... it definitely stored mine!

Detoxification of Internal Organs

An crucial contributor to how I cured my breast most cancers obviously become via the procedure of cleansing positive organs, specially the liver, kidneys, and lymphatic systems. My holistic practitioner had me observe a positive protocol that I can percentage part of with you to provide you a few perception. (Unfortunately, because of felony motives I can't absolutely reveal the names of all the goods I used to aid the cleansing procedure.) Focusing on cleansing your frame is a non-public act of self-care because it takes more time, attention and attempt to your everyday existence. It isn't always an clean component to experience. However, it's miles tremendously beneficial. I nonetheless have a few detox protocols that I often have interaction in in order that my frame keeps to live as healthful as possible, and maintain disorder away.

The purpose of cleansing become to dispose of constructed up pollution and extra mucus from my machine in order that my frame ought to greater correctly heal itself. The complete protocol lasted numerous days, and I become bowled over as to how an awful lot junk and gunk got here out of my frame close to the stop of the time. It actually felt like I had an earthquake internal me and I sincerely ended up dropping 5 pounds! I had buddies who had comparable reports so I become now no longer concerned approximately the type of results it become having on my frame. One of the maximum crucial matters is to drink lots of water with a view to assist the pollution flush nicely and correctly out of your frame.

The first organ I specially detoxed become my liver, as it's miles critical for cleansing your blood. The protocol my holistic practitioner furnished me become quite straightforward. I become to consume a breakfast and lunch that contained NO FATS whatsoever (no olive oil, no butter, no nuts), and prevent all consuming through 2pm.

I become then requested to observe this unique liver cleaning recipe of substances and timeline with a view to correctly spark off my liver.

Ingredients needed:

- 4 tablespoons of Epsom salt
- 2 red grapefruits
- 4 ounces (½ cup) extra virgin cold pressed olive oil
- 3 cups distilled water

6:00pm

- Mix 4 tablespoons of Epsom salt in 3 cups distilled water
- Drink ¾ Epsom salts mixture

8:00pm

- Drink ¾ cup Epsom salts mixture

9:30pm

- Squeeze the 2 red grapefruits by hand, remove pulp.
- Measure 2/3 cup of the juice and place into a bottle with a lid.
- Add to this 4-ounce extra virgin cold pressed olive oil and cover.
- Shake the contents the mixture vigorously to ensure ingredients thoroughly mixed together

10:00pm

- Walk to your bedside and while standing, drink all of the olive oil/grape mixture within 5 minutes.
- Lie on your back, head high on your pillow… stay in this position until yo asleep. If you have to get up to go to the bathroom, go back to bed after. Lying on the back is important for the liver cleanse.

In the morning, it's miles crucial which you observe those steps:

6:30am

- Drink ¾ cup Epsom salt mixture

8:30am

- Drink ¾ cup Epsom salt mixture

10:30am
- Drink 1 cup of juice (any 100% juice, no sugar added, not from concentr

12:00pm
- Eat a piece of fruit (any variety, whole)

I hold to often exercise one-of-a-kind cleansing approaches even now that I am most cancers-free. I keep it as an crucial a part of selfcare practices. It makes me experience first rate and I consider it like a type of music up for my frame.

Keeping a Gratitude Journal

The past due Dr. Maya Angelou said:

"If you do now no longer like some thing, alternate it.
If you can't alternate it, alternate the manner you consider it."

I want to maintain this concept near as I navigate existence. Especially after I am experiencing hardships. One of my mentors as soon as recommended me that with a view to gather whatever of fee, I ought to first display gratitude. This honestly struck me as I had now no longer idea approximately my existence like that before.

My non-public mirrored image on gratitude is that we do now no longer recognize what we've till we've misplaced it. Connecting to gratitude is a effective manner that you may hook up with your existence.

If you aren't acquainted with precisely what a gratitude magazine is, allow me offer a few perception and a leaping off factor for you. You can use a diary or pocket book of a few sort. In it you may mirror on stuff you are thankful for. It may be any and all matters... anything is inspiring you that day! Perhaps you're thankful for the smooth air to respire or the smooth walking water you've got got get right of entry to to. Perhaps you hook up with matters which are greater non-public to you. This is a non-public gratitude magazine simply a good way to each hook up with the riches of your existence withinside the second in addition to some thing that you could want to refer returned on as a reflective exercise.

Gratitude journals sincerely keep a whole lot of electricity and advantages which could upload a whole lot of fee for your existence. A image of those advantages include:
- Better psychological and physical health
- Experiencing more empathy and less aggressive feelings towards others
- Greater mental strength
- Better sleep
- Become more resilient in your life
- Experience more experience creativity
- ...and more!

(Source: Lauren Jessen, The Benefits of a Gratitude Journal)

Listen to Relaxing Music

Music is frequently called an global language. It is a language with out words, however is conversation via Sound! When I become deep withinside the procedure of recovery my most cancers, my holistic health practitioner recommended me to keep away from setting myself in any annoying situations. This is because of the reality that one of the reasons of most cancers is continual stress. So, I needed to be very conscious of what environments I become growing round myself.

I became to tune to assist create greater enjoyable recovery areas in my lifestyles. Because of now no longer looking to set off strain I became very unique of the tune I chose. For me, classical and gospel tune make me sense comfortable and at ease. Some of my preferred classical portions consist of Water Music through Handel, and some thing this is piano based. If you aren't acquainted with gospel tune, it's far a style of Christian tune that I individually discover very soothing.

What form of tune makes you sense calmer and greater grounded? It is a laugh to test and find out what makes you sense excellent. You can use the tune which you pick to shift you right into a calmer nation whilst you want it. You can play it at precise instances of your day, or possibly use it as a device to apply whilst you sense your strain tiers rising. However you operate it, be open to connecting to the strength of tune as a manner that will help you heal and preserve you healthful.

Have a Laugh!

I am certain you've got got heard the vintage adage "Laughter is the excellent medicine!" Laughter has great recovery homes for the frame. I as soon as study approximately a person who after an extended war of most cancers became given only some months to live. He determined to observe comedy suggests all day lengthy so as to hook up with laughter and convey greater pleasure into what became prepurported to be darker days. I am now no longer certain clearly the way it happened, however the guy did now no longer die from his infection and survived his diagnosis.

There are incredible noted health benefits of laughter:
- It fortifies your immune system
- It helps you feel less pain (both physically and emotionally)
- It can increase blood flow through the body, most specifically to the hea
- It is shown to reduce inflammation
- It can help reduce anxiety and boost your mood in a more positive way
- Laughter helps you make it through tough times
- …. and much more!

(Source: "20 Crazy Health Benefits of Laughter-No Joke" Tehrene Firman, July 26, 2018)

I needed to determine out a manner to convey greater laughter into my lifestyles. The first component I did became enroll in an e mail carrier that despatched a funny story every day to my
inbox. What a satisfaction it's far to obtain a funny story in my inbox each morning! It offers me some thing to grin approximately earlier than I ought

to consider the greater severe matters in my lifestyles.

I additionally volunteered for the function of "Joke Master" at some point of my time with Toastmasters. As I formerly mentioned, Toastmasters International is an worldwide affiliation in which humans sign up to enhance on their communication, management and presentation skills.

While in Toastmasters there are one of a kind membership roles that one may also take on, with one in all them being the "Joke Master" or stand-up comedian of your membership. Essentially I normally volunteered to percentage jokes so that you can lighten the temper of meetings. Cracking jokes truly made me sense much less strain and anxiety, and I ought to sincerely see the way it made different participants sense at ease. I clearly loved my time in that position!

I wish which you are stimulated to dive deeper into your very own self-care practices. If up till this factor on your lifestyles you haven't clearly idea approximately it, I wish which you pass ahead and discover approaches to make self-care a part of your every day lifestyles.

Beyond self-care there may be any other layer of looking after your self and persevering with to construct upon that basis that we spoke of. Have you ever thought about ways that you can "fertilize" your body with more energy and life force? I want to talk about it a bit deeper so that you may gain insight as to how you can apply these incredible practices yourself and take good care.

Chapter 8

"Fertilize" Your Body

"A healthful life-style consists of exercise, nutrition, healthful sleep styles and a healthful organization of friends."
— Sophie Grégoire Trudeau

8

I love that quote as it constantly rings a bell in my memory that there may be a controversy for the easy matters. This subsequent layer of your health adventure is going past self- care. It is all approximately locating matters similarly to the entirety we've got pointed out so as to create a well "fertilized" frame which can keep to help your boom and the first rate fitness you've got got found. Your adventure to conquering most cancers or stopping it's far multifaceted. I need to percentage a few matters I sense are greater diffused and had been delivered to my ordinary as soon as I had hooked up the muse of my protocols. You can take those in your very own, or possibly they'll encourage you to get curious approximately your very own specific approaches of fertilizing your very own frame. Find what works for you!

Soak Up the Sun

It is of extreme significance to get sufficient solar. Sunshine triggers manufacturing of Vitamin D, that is an vital nutrient wanted withinside the frame. (I spoke approximately this in Chapter 4.) However, did you realize that sitting withinside the sunshine also can assist you with a lot greater? Think approximately it. I am certain that there are instances in which you've got got evidently craved feeling the solar for your pores and skin or face. Perhaps it became after an extended winter (if withinside the northern hemisphere). Perhaps after a stretch of wet days.

As humans, we're obviously drawn to the sunshine! Its fitness advantages certainly is aware of no bounds:

- It boosts your mood

- Reduces stress and pain associated with surgery

- Builds the immune system

- It can reduce cancer risks (because of the Vitamin D that it will natu produce on your frame)

- Naturally kills bad bacteria

- and more!

(Source: Hamilton Recruitment: Caribbean & Bermuda Jobs)

How do you typically get a few sunshine? I will take the time to take a seat down out on my balcony or cross for a stroll with the aim to definitely absorb the solar. I actually have additionally were given into the addiction of parking a piece in addition from entrances once I am out and approximately in order that I can also additionally get a few solar whilst taking walks to the door of a store or business. These are clean approaches to contain greater solar into your time table whilst you cross approximately your every day business.

When I turned into first discussing this with my holistic physician, she added up the truth that darkish skinned humans (as I am) want greater sunshine than caucasian individuals. This is as it takes longer for darkish skinned humans to fabricate and synthesize the solar into Vitamin D. On pinnacle of this I should be greater conscious due to the fact I stay in Canada, so the quantity of direct solar I can certainly acquire is pretty much less in comparison to whilst residing in tropical countries.

When you decide to spending time withinside the solar, you now no longer handiest substantially have an effect on your bodily fitness however you fertilize incredible matters for all elements of you. Getting solar is multidimensional in its restoration homes.

Drinking My "Daily Concoction"

As mentioned in Chapter 3, garlic and lemons each have incredible dietary value. Another manner that I improve my consumption of those potent, restoration ingredients is to drink 1.five oz of a mix of natural garlic and natural lemon. My physician advocated this type of "fitness shot" as a manner to growth my consumption of the excellent advantages of the garlic and lemon combined. Of course, this concoction isn't always for the faint of heart! The scent and flavor are pretty stinky and in case you aren't used to it, it can take the time to adapt.

However, as with something new, addiction or ordinary, you surely do get used to it! I actually have certainly come to experience this a part of my every day ordinary as I can surely hook up with the excellent restoration homes that I am installing my frame to my excessive stage of bodily fitness.

Why garlic and lemon together? Well, first off the flavor is certainly pretty nice. I am certain you might imagine of Some dishes in which garlic and lemon are used to create a few extraordinary tasting food. So, it could be visible as a taste shot. We extensively included the fitness advantages of garlic. In addition to matters mentioned, the sulphureous compounds in garlic are in which the most cancers combating magic lies. These specific compounds were studied for his or her cappotential to inhibit cancerous cells and block tumors with the aid of using slowing DNA replication. Incredible! Adding the energy of lemon on pinnacle of that certainly takes it to the following stage. Not handiest does lemon have severa fitness advantages starting from handling high blood pressure to helping in weight loss, it's been observed to assist kill most cancers cells. (Source: The Benefits and Uses for Lemon Juice for Cancer with the aid of using Dr Maria. Health and Wellness, May five, 2018) According to a look at posted in 2016 on nutrients, lemons have anticancer advantages for prostate, breast, stomach, liver, cervix, pancreas and colon most cancers cells. It is vital to word that those findings are from managed research on most cancers cells in a lab.

(Source: Lemons and most cancers: Are they protective? Livestrong.com)

Drinking this shot of garlic and lemon each day makes me experience revitalized and linked to my bodily fitness. It is an concept now no longer for everyone, however I needed to proportion it because it makes me experience extraordinary. It surely turned into a sport changer.

Enjoying Fresh Fruit and Vegetable Smoothies

A fantastic way to ensure you are getting enough of the various fruits and vegetables that are important to eat when looking to prevent or fight cancer is to drink them! Smoothies are drinks made with blended fruits and vegetables, and a high-quality manner to contain greater powerful, uncooked ingredients into your diet.

I love all smoothie flavors and certainly do now no longer have a favorite one. I did now no longer assume to drink them earlier than my holistic practitioner advocated them due to their fitness advantages. Now I typically experience them on weekends for breakfast once I am now no longer training intermittent fasting. I observed that after I began out ingesting smoothies, they gave me a heightened experience of well-being! I'm guessing it's miles from all of the extraordinary substances packed into one drink!

The advantages of ingesting clean smoothies are plentiful:

- Because of the high-water content in the fruits and vegetables, they help prevent dehydration

- Controls mood swings and helps fight depression

- They are a high dose of good fiber

- Assists in detoxing the body

- May balance hormonal functioning

- A great source of antioxidants which can help keep in check the grow free radicals and other cancer-causing agents

- Depending on ingredients, will reduce the chance of cancers (exa broccoli and cauliflower are fantastic cancer fighting ingredients you easily add to your smoothies)

- ... and more!

(Source: https://easyhealthysmoothie.com)

Incorporating smoothies into my recurring is this sort of adorable ritual for me. Again, I recognise that I am taking the time to do some thing excellent for my frame. But it is going past simply the ingredients. Making and ingesting smoothies has emerge as a ritual that now no longer simplest nourishes my frame however additionally my mind. It asks me to take a ruin in my day and do some thing excellent for myself.

Hydrate! Hydrate! Hydrate!

When I started my most cancers combating journey, I were advised via way of means of numerous docs that I changed into now no longer ingesting sufficient water. I admit, ingesting sufficient water and staying hydrated changed into now no longer truly on my radar whilst it got here to considering my fitness. But given that I started the method of cleansing my inner organs and switching my recognition to residing a lifestyles in which I am in excellent fitness, ingesting sufficient water has actually emerge as a priority. You may also have the equal war with regards to ingesting sufficient water, however as soon as you exchange some behavior it isn't as difficult as you suppose.

Upon waking withinside the morning, the primary aspect I do is drink a pitcher of water. I normally hold a pitcher of water on my night time stand in case I experience thirsty at Some point of the night time. If I do now no longer drink it then, it's miles already awaiting me once I wake up! I take the time to drink a pitcher of water round my food in place of with my meals. I locate this is extra powerful in truly hydrating me. So, I will generally tend to drink a pitcher of water half-hour earlier than eating, then additionally wait till half-hour after to have a pitcher. Another new addiction that I now have is maintaining a bottle of water in my handbag in any respect times. It is then effectively to be had to sip on once I am using somewhere, or once I am out and approximately strolling errands. It is truly crucial to have water without delay to be had while you are thirsty. Essentially continually hold a few water close by and start noticing while you are thirsty, or simply get into the addiction of continually sipping your water. It turns into some thing which you not should suppose approximately.

A simple way I learned to determine if I am drinking enough water and staying hydrated throughout my day is to examine my urine when I go to the washroom. This is one of the simplest ways of knowing if you need to be drinking more water, even if you are not necessarily thirsty. If the color of your urine is dark yellow, this is an indication of being dehydrated. If it is pale yellow in color, then you are drinking enough water. This is a quick and easy way to take stock of your hydration level. If you wish to have more of an actual calculation, it is easy to predetermine the ideal amount of water you should be drinking in a day. Take your weight in pounds and divide it into two, and that is the number of ounces of water you should be consuming in a day. For example, if you weigh 150 pounds, half of that is 75, so your daily intake of water with that weight would be 75 ounces of water.

The nice of the water you're ingesting is crucial. I continually boil my water first after which use a popular filter. I additionally hold my water in a vessel at room temperature. I locate my tooth are too touchy to drink bloodless things. (Sometimes I will also upload a few lemon slices, flaxseed or apple cider vinegar to make my water extra flavorful!) However, a few additionally experience that ingesting bloodless water may be negative for your fitness. I don't forget once I lived in Asia, I observed nobody drank bloodless liquids with any in their food. They rather selected warm soup or tea. Of course, that is very exceptional from popular North American practices. People there might inform me that ailments might be cured via way of means of ingesting warm liquids. They additionally expressed that they believed humans withinside the western international locations suffered from clogged arteries due to the fact they ate warm meals with bloodless water... What an thrilling perspective!

When I am hydrated, I experience excellent. I even have discovered that staying hydrated truly continues my head clear, and I am capable of live inspired and focused. I can not trust that it changed into now no longer till my fitness failed that I truly paid interest to my water consumption. If you already drink sufficient water, excellent for you! If now no longer, I urge you to begin these days to create this new addiction.

Find Health Specialists to Work With

You can not do it alone. No remember how tough you attempt a good way to advantage choicest fitness I assume it's far honestly vital to discover extraordinary fitness practitioners which you need to interact with to make your closing fitness team. After my most cancers diagnosis, it have become crucial to go to my holistic medical doctor as soon as a month or each different month a good way to maintain up with the extraordinary protocols that had been vital as I opted out of chemotherapy treatment. It turned into fantastic to the touch base with a person who I knew desired to assist me and had my first-rate hobby at heart. I found out a lot from her and knew I ought to anticipate her assist via that hard time.

If you discover you need to control whatever fitness wise, be it acute or chronic, minor or serious, there are experts in each unmarried discipline geared up to assist you. I sense that is an vital a part of your dedication to "fertilize" your frame properly so you may also develop your potential. There aren't anyt any limits to what this may appear to be for your existence. However, you can not cross it alone. Trust me. Find the assist you want after which watch your self develop and achieve something you placed your thoughts to! I continue to be all the time thankful to my holistic medical doctor for assisting me overcome my breast most cancers, and coaching me a way to keep helping my fitness a good way to stay most cancers-free.

I wish which you see the extraordinary approaches wherein you could assist your self to create a fertile existence wherein you could thrive and attain your fitness goals. Never overlook that each unmarried component you decide to can and could assist you withinside the lengthy run.

I even have in brief touched upon the non secular factor of recuperation in preceding chapters. However, it's far now time to do a deeper dive. I need to proportion with you the way maintaining the religion and having wish performed crucial roles in my most cancers adventure.

Chapter 9

The Power of Faith and Hope

> *"Be devoted in small matters due to the fact it's far in them that your energy lies."*
> — Mother Teresa

9

An vital factor of my recuperation adventure while not having to apply chemotherapy turned into committing to have a more potent, greater vertical fellowship with God. I had usually been a devoted man or woman however after I turned into confronted with the information of my most cancers diagnosis, I needed to take a step again and begin honestly analyzing what turned into vital to me. The manner I have been residing my existence up till that factor turned into in keeping with my religion however I knew that if I made a brand new dedication my recuperation adventure could be infused with greater mild and wish.

The Bible states: "But Jesus checked out them and said, "With guy that is impossible, however with God all matters are possible." {Matthew 19:26} Let me show you how I developed a stronger relationship with God and how it brought much inspiration to my life.

Daily Morning Devotionals

What in case you commenced your day via way of means of taking a couple of minutes to take a seat down and hook up with some thing this is extra than your self? This is wherein day by day devotionals can assist. Daily devotionals are Christian spiritual courses that offer particular non secular readings for every calendar day. They are both posted as a month-to-month or every year collection.

First and foremost, after I awaken the primary component, I say to start out my day is: "Good morning Holy Spirit, thanks for waking me up from sleep!"

I by no means need to take without any consideration the reality that I honestly awoke and I am alive to stay some other day. I then circulate to study the devotional. I open up the web page that corresponds to the date and make an effort to study what's offered. The codecs are reflections or quick prayers, and feature a corresponding biblical reference. There is usually a fantastic uplifting identify in order to come up with an concept of the subject of the day. Here are a few examples:

- Your Root is Growing Strong, Never Quit Now!
- The Secret of Shutting the Door
- There is a Minstrel in You!
- Faith-Building Memories
- I am an Eagle and Not a Grasshopper
- The Power of Prayer
- and many more…..

(Source: Our Daily Manna: A Daily Devotional Booklet for Champions July to September 2021)

Devotionals are exceedingly useful for your existence. By imparting God your devotion, you could get hold of steering in return. You get to now no longer best understand your self better, however additionally increase a more potent courting with Jesus, in addition to the Holy Spirit. In our crazy, fast moving international it provides an possibility to take a seat down still. It is likewise a wonderful manner to deliver your own circle of relatives and cherished ones collectively and create a deeper private courting with them. All in all, devotionals are a fantastic manner to assist control stress, that you clearly understand is vital to steer a more healthy existence. (Source: Call to Glory, an independent, essential Baptist, king James Devotional)

I discover devotionals very positive, thought-scary and uplifting. After taking time to study them, I sense geared up to address my day with gusto! Devotionals assist beef up all components of me: spiritually, bodily and mentally. This in flip no question allows beef up my immune device and allows save you illness.

Listen to Gospel and Classical Music

As I formerly noted, I love lifting my spirits through being attentive to gospel and classical track. I even have constantly had an appreciation for classical track
seeing that I turned into younger. (I want I by no means gave up mastering to play the piano!) These genres of track maintain me feeling comfortable and grounded.

Gospel track specially is a kind of Christian track this is very devotional to God, Jesus and the Holy Spirit. This track promotes religion and conjures up the soul. I will actually pay attention to it during my complete day: once I am withinside the shower, taking a walk, withinside the car… anywhere! It allows me do not forget the greater essential matters in life.

Gospel track has been observed to offer human beings a experience of purpose (source: Abbey Cheche, Arts and Entertainment, April 18, 2018) When you're withinside the center of recuperation your self from most cancers or coping with another fitness issues, it's miles vital to have a experience of some thing larger and higher coming your manner. It can instill a experience of desire for the times ahead.

Classical track has constantly been visible as a high-quality device to apply in human beings's recuperation processes. Whether it's coping with pain, enhancing sleep or stronger intellectual alertness, this kind of track may be tremendous to attain for withinside the center of a recuperation adventure or to maintain ailment at bay. (Source: Shari Mathias, Parker Symphony Orchestra)

As I went via my very own recuperation adventure, each gospel and classical track helped me loosen up and at instances take me away to a one of a kind location; an area wherein I turned into very healthful and felt incredible. Again, those track genres have been capable of assist me maintain my religion, even on darker days. It helped me continue to be grounded and centered at the brighter days ahead.

Daily Intercessory Prayer

If you aren't acquainted with it, intercessory prayer is praying on behalf of others or for the desires of others. It is a one of a kind manner of connecting to praying to God as your prayers are centered on others. For example, the week's agenda for my organization can also additionally seem like this:

- Monday we pray for each other's family
- Tuesday we pray for our pastors
- Wednesday we pray for government leaders
- Thursday we pray for students
- Friday we pray for business owners
- Saturday we pray for teachers

As I noted in Chapter 6, I sense blessed to be a part of a prayer and Bible examine organization that meets every day. We have all devoted to be at the phone from 6-6:30am (or till 7am Saturday). We have a agenda wherein we consciously pray for human beings withinside the organization. We are seven participants and of the identical participants are scheduled to desire on Mondays and Wednesdays; others are scheduled to hope on Tuesdays and Thursdays. Two are scheduled to guide prayers on Thursdays; others on Fridays and on Saturdays. We have Sunday off to sleep in. The pastor can even have a subject for every day, for which he'll provide his very own mirrored image on in addition to scriptures from the Bible. Topics can also additionally consist of things like anger, recuperation, righteousness, grace, hope, and kindness.

I pray continuously and sense prayer can provide a lot to the individual:

- A better sense of self
- Good for your heart
- Increases life span
- Improves attitude
- Gain forgiveness

- Relieves stress
- Maintain a positive outlook on life
- Recovery: "After a situation leaves you emotionally or physically distra recovery is a timely process. Prayer serves as a way to deal with aftermath and keep one's faith. Your body and mind are focused sole healing while prayer keeps you centered and hopeful."

(Source: Top 10 Health Benefits of Praying through Health Fitness Revolution, May 21, 2015)

My prayer organization presented me their very own prayers on a every day basis, and this turned into a part of the purpose I healed.

Reading From the Bible Daily

If you need to reinforce your pleasure and boom your typical awareness, studying from the Bible every day may be a effective device. I noted that, as a part of my prayer organization, we study scripture every day. I love while it's miles my flip to proportion the effective phrases of God with my friends. Starting the day this manner constantly offers me a tremendous enhance of suggestion and propels me ahead to have a effective day.

Reading the Bible is a wealthy and gratifying experience. It pleases God while you hook up with those effective phrases and brings you towards Divinity. Doesn't that sound like a pleasing location to be?

Sit in a "Thinking" Chair

I am certain it's miles turning into clean that I even have a normal morning ordinary that allows me hook up with God and my religion. Another lovable component I do every morning is make the effort to take a seat down in my Thinking Chair. I discovered this workout from one in all my mentors years ago.

As a part of your morning devotional time, you virtually take a seat down and think. Make certain the chair is comfortable. Perhaps it's miles in a pleasing place of your home. You virtually make the effort to take a seat

down, be quiet and think. It is a private workout that you could make your very own. During my time in my Thinking Chair, I want to focus
On how I can higher all of the aspects of my lifestyles: spiritual, financial, physical, social, emotional and mental. Sometimes I stroll away simply having loved connecting with my thoughts. Sometimes I stroll away with a tremendous concept or a solution to a trouble that desires to be solved. In any regard, it's miles in no way wasted time.

A large a part of enhancing my lifestyles is likewise how I can be of carrier to others.
Motivational speaker Zig Ziglar said:

"If you assist sufficient humans get what they need, you'll get what you need."

I take this to heart, and produce a variety of awareness to being of advantage to others. It changed into particularly useful for the duration of the time even as I changed into combating my breast most cancers. It helped me take awareness from myself and location it on others, which felt good. It jogged my memory that there has been extra to my lifestyles than simply my most cancers adventure.

I had masses of notable moments in my Thinking Chair, and might in no way pass over my session. Even once I am pressed for time, I will nonetheless usually take as a minimum a couple of minutes to simply stop, and think.

When I decide to starting every day with my morning devotion, it offers me the religion and desire to triumph over all adversities I may also face now and withinside the future. While I changed into coping with my most cancers recuperation it changed into sincerely essential to deepen my connection to God in any manner I may want to. Having religion in a better energy helped me grow to be steadfast, and at once performed a component in conquering my breast most cancers, no doubt!

I additionally had an awesome assist circle of buddies and own circle of relatives praying for me, and maintaining the religion that I might come thru the alternative facet. Even my personal pastor, upon locating out approximately my diagnosis, declared that I might now no longer die, and might stay to percentage my testimony. (And right here I am scripting this book!)

Keeping desire alive inside your self and surrounding your self with folks who consider in you is powerful. There are research accessible which nation that individuals who had been positive for the duration of their ailments were given higher quicker than individuals who had been negative:

"For decades, many researchers idea the improve in immunity changed into due to the truth that positive humans had been much more likely to attend to their fitness. But extra latest research have proven that a hopeful outlook is clearly what affects immunity. Looking on the intense facet makes you much less in all likelihood to get a chilly or contamination due to the fact optimism maintains your immune device acting at its peak." (Source: 7 Ways to heal your frame with the aid of using the use of the energy of your mind, subsidized with the aid of using technology with the aid of using Amy Morin) Remaining hopeful and high quality changed into a part of what stored me.

Because of my warfare with breast most cancers, my lifestyles modified for the higher. Some of those modifications had been large and a few had been subtle. Let me percentage with you what my lifestyles gave the look of and felt like when I changed into identified and cured. I am all the time modified and might in no way alternate my enjoy for anything.

Chapter 10

My Life After Breast Cancer

"A man's legacy is decided with the aid of using how the tale ends."
— Leonardo DiCaprio

10

Because of my breast most cancers adventure, my lifestyles without a doubt modified dramatically. Now that I am lower back to complete fitness after beating the most cancers naturally, I can genuinely see what a blessing in conceal that adventure changed into. My lifestyles is all the time modified for the higher and I will all the time be glad about what I actually have learned.

I need to percentage with you a few reflections on how I experience now, the modifications I skilled and invite you to mirror on how you can keep growing and increase your personal lifestyles. Even in case you are going thru your personal struggles or challenges, lifestyles has a lot to provide you in go back for you attempting new matters or displaying up extra than ever before.

Give More, Appreciate Life More

As I referred to before, even as I changed into present process my recuperation to higher fitness, I changed into invited to assist feed the homeless and much less privileged each Sunday with a few individuals from my Bible observe group. My attitude on how I engage with my network modified dramatically for the duration of that time. I may want to genuinely experience that the extra I changed into inclined to give, the extra I preferred all of the goodness in my personal lifestyles.

It is a strong team of five people and we manage to feed about 50-80 homeless people every Sunday in downtown Toronto. I find it distressing that I live in a rich country such as Canada and there are people who do not have food to eat. I have met many of these less fortunate people and am grateful, as I doubt I would have crossed paths with them otherwise.

Creating a dating with this network thru our efforts each Sunday makes me sense like I am giving again in a few small manner. In turn, it makes my very own lifestyles sense even extra wealthy and fulfilling.

Connect to Even More Gratitude

As I cited earlier than, having an mind-set of gratitude is an critical a part of a restoration adventure. It continues you linked to the larger picture. I keep to preserve a gratitude magazine to this day. I make an effort to jot down in it each night time earlier than I visit bed. It continually makes me sense calm and much less careworn earlier than I near my eyes for the night time. Keeping up with my gratitude practices has additionally allowed me to in addition study plenty approximately myself, and heightens my self-awareness. I additionally love having a file of reflections that I can refer again to once I want a strong reminder of all of the top in my lifestyles.

I observed that when incorporating a aware gratitude exercise I actually have a miles more appreciation for the finer matters in lifestyles. As well, I can without problems see extra possibilities to percentage my riches whilst top matters come into my lifestyles. Perspective is the entirety in relation to being thankful for what you have.

Self-Improvement

I actually have continually been a curious character and dedicated to growth. However, I determined that in my most cancers adventure I commenced to position greater recognition on my lifestyles outdoor of labor and commenced seeing my lifestyles with a broader lens. The approaches I interact with my very own self-development multiplied and nevertheless are with me today. Let me in brief percentage with you a few highlights in desire that it could encourage you to preserve developing and committing to some thing extra on your lifestyles.

Read More Books

One of my mentors continually said "Readers are leaders." After I conquered my breast most cancers, I determined that I commenced studying plenty extra than usual. Of route, we have been all at domestic extra due to the pandemic. However, I couldn't get sufficient of studying

self-improvement books and have become involved as to how I ought to exceptional use this lifestyles that were talented to me. (This additionally caused attending extra on-line instructions and seminars, all with makes a speciality of self-development.) Making studying part of your regular lifestyles is exceptionally useful on your average fitness. Beyond enhancing your brain
connectivity and stopping cognitive decline, studying has been proven to decrease your coronary heart charge and blood stress and assist combat depression (source: Rebecca Joy Stanborough, MFA October 15, 2019)

If you already do now no longer have a robust dating with studying, I urge you to discover the time and make it happen. You will observe a distinction on your lifestyles.

Take Online Courses

As I cited above, I determined myself taking extra on-line publications. Of route, all through the pandemic the entirety moved to digital platforms. But this changed into this kind of gift! Suddenly I ought to take instructions and publications that have been now no longer to be had to me earlier than they went on-line. Some have been unfastened and a few I actually made the economic funding in once I felt it to be of value. To be honest, I honestly loved taking instructions on-line withinside the consolation of my very own domestic. It makes me sense much less careworn and extra comfortable.

Eating Well

When I commenced converting my consuming conduct all through my adventure to triumph over most cancers, my holistic health practitioner continually jogged my memory to "Let meals be thy medicinal drug and allow medicinal drug be thy meals." (Source: Hippocrates, Greek Physician.) By this adage, Hippocrates changed into emphasizing the significance of vitamins to save you or treatment disease. Learning extra approximately how meals affected my fitness brought about me to make many adjustments to my diet, lots of which I nevertheless exercise today. Sometimes it may be complicated in my non-public lifestyles as I should decline social invites at times. However, I could by no means alternate the manner I now sense for anything.

Managing Stress

In our present day world, there may be no manner to break out strain altogether. However, over the route of my restoration adventure it have become very clean to me the significance of coping with strain on your lifestyles and coping with it well.

As I cited at the start of the ee-e book, one of the viable reasons of most cancers is strain. This is due to the consequences of strain at the frame. At the time of publishing this ee-e book I am reading to grow to be an authorized fitness and lifestyles teach and, all through my studies, the approaches wherein strain negatively influences the frame has arise severa times.

The listing is pretty extensive, however allow me percentage some highlights with you:

- Increases inflammation in the body which can be the basis for many dise
- Causes a lowering of levels in growth hormones which are essen healing, rebuilding and growing all tissues in the body
- Increases resistance to insulin, resulting in diabetes, heart disease weight gain
- Decreases nutrient absorption and increase nutrient excretion
- Decreases sex hormones, resulting in a decrease in muscle mass or lowe drive

(Source: The Effects of Stress at the Body, Health Coach Institute)

I ought to pass on. I am certain this image offers you a experience of ways strain infiltrates all structures in our frame and reasons first-rate harm.

In order to manipulate pressure, there are numerous methods you may technique it, and plenty of sports you may do. The following are what works thoroughly for me, that I consist of frequently in my days which will preserve my pressure in check.

Take Naps - Every day I take time for a "siesta" that's a day nap. I intention for thirty minutes; however, every now and then that modifications relying on my agenda for the day. These days I specially make money working from home so becoming in a sleep is plenty easier. Taking time each day for important relaxation, be it a sleep or otherwise, may be very strengthening to your immune system. There are a few businesses consisting of Google that have sound asleep pods that they inspire their personnel to use, and take twenty minute strength naps which will stay
rejuvenated and energized.

Daily Walk - Every day I cross for a brisk stroll. If I can, I will attempt to get it in in the course of the morning to present myself an lively boost. I take the time to preserve a brisk tempo and additionally swing my hands which will get my coronary heart charge up. My day by day stroll lightens my temper and feels energizing! It offers me a extra high-quality outlook on my day. I certainly word a distinction in my thoughts and frame once I can not match it in.

Breathe Deeply - Breathing deeply is every other manner I convey matters again into focus, with the intention to speak. It facilitates me get gift and makes my thoughts experience extra clean and at ease. There is a method that I frequently use, particularly if I am feeling a piece better degree of pressure than usual. It is referred to as the field respiratory approach or rectangular respiratory. What you do is consciously convey your breath into 4 parts. You can attempt it proper now with me. Inhale deeply into your stomach for 4 counts. Gently keep the breath for 4 counts. Slowly exhale the breath for 4 counts and keep the breath out for 4 counts. Continue this breath cycle for so long as is required. It is an first-rate device which can make your thoughts experience extra focused very quick.

Get a Massage - I commenced getting everyday massages after my lumpectomy that I acquired proper after my most cancers diagnosis. I certainly observed the high-quality consequences in my existence so I actually have selected to preserve massages as part of my everyday routine. They assist me experience extra rejuvenated and nearly like a brand new person! It may be very effective how plenty getting a rub down can shift your attitude and outlook.

Comedies, Movies and Sermons

After recuperation from this dreadful disease, I now will constantly make time to have a laugh, watch a movie and connect to God. I actually have noted all the above in the course of the direction of the ee-e book. But I am highlighting them one extra time due to the fact that is how critical they nonetheless are to me.

I love looking comedy shows, from tv collection to rise up specials. They in no way stop to simply make me experience higher once I want a "pick me up." I love that I can activate my tv and some thing can provide the medication of laughter so quick to me. The equal with looking a movie. Movies are a risk to break out your personal existence for a while, however I constantly come away feeling like I discovered some thing approximately people or myself. Storytelling withinside the shape of a movie is a completely effective manner to hook up with matters which are outdoor of your world. In addition to Hollywood films, I additionally love looking Bollywood and Nollywood.

In phrases of enticing with sermons, we're so fortunate now as there are numerous sermons to be had on line and on tv. I can both simply song in and be reminded of God's effective phrases and teachings, or I can particularly searching for out a sermon that I want to hear. They constantly assist me stay found in my personal existence and join deeply to what certainly matters.

My existence after conquering most cancers feels complete and exciting. I experience thankful that I went thru my experience. No count how tough demanding situations appeared on the time, I can now see the way it changed into all really well worth it. Today, I experience like a extra entire person, and all of the training I discovered had been invaluable.

This adventure has been so inspiring in fact, that I determined to sign up and end up an authorized fitness and existence coach. Even starting to write this ee-e book solidified for me that I need to preserve to assist human beings of their personal fitness the excellent I can. Let us all take into account that fitness is wealth. There is constantly mild on the cease of the tunnel!

Printed in Great Britain
by Amazon